Unless Recalled Earlier

ATTITUDES ON ALTITUDE

ATTITUDES

ON

ALTITUDE

Pioneers of Medical Research in Colorado's High Mountains

———— Edited by ————

John T. Reeves and Robert F. Grover

University Press of Colorado

© 2001 by the University Press of Colorado
International Standard Book Number 0-87081-645-4

Published by the University Press of Colorado
5589 Arapahoe Avenue, Suite 206C
Boulder, Colorado 80303

The University Press of Colorado is a cooperative publishing enterprise supported, in part, by
Adams State College, Colorado State University, Fort Lewis College, Mesa State College,
Metropolitan State College of Denver, University of Colorado, University of Northern
Colorado, University of Southern Colorado, and Western State College of Colorado.

The paper used in this publication meets the minimum requirements of the American National
Standard for Information Sciences—Permanence of Paper for Printed Library Materials. ANSI
Z39.48-1992

Library of Congress Cataloging-in-Publication Data

Attitudes on altitude : pioneers of medical research in Colorado's high mountains / Editors,
John T. Reeves, M.D. and Robert F. Grover.
    p. cm.
  Includes bibliographical references and index.
  ISBN 0-87081-645-4 (hbk. : alk. paper)
  1. Altitude, Influence of—Research—Colorado—History. 2. Mountain sickness—Research—
Colorado—History. I. Reeves, John T. II. Grover, Robert F., 1924–

  QP82.2.A4 A88 2001
  616.9'893—dc21

                                                              2001002739

Design by Daniel Pratt

10 09 08 07 06 05 04 03 02 01   10 9 8 7 6 5 4 3 2 1

To the memory of
Estelle B. Grover,
partner, companion, friend, collaborator,
who suggested the title
for this volume,

And in dedication to the patience of
Carol S. Reeves

CONTENTS

ILLUSTRATIONS

Table

PREFACE

Having spent more than four decades in high-altitude research in Colorado, we, the editors, wanted to pay homage to those who went before us, those who laid the foundations for subsequent work at altitudes. We have selected for presentation seven episodes where all of the participants were pioneers who made important and novel contributions to health at high altitude within Colorado. Of course we wanted to show why their work was important, why Colorado was important, and why they did what they did. And, even more, we wanted to illuminate the pioneers themselves, their lives, their motives, their successes, and their failures. Who should write these stories? Should we do it all or should we call in a different expert to write each chapter?

When we began more than ten years ago, our colleagues gave us conflicting advice. With multiple experts, some said, the book would be more authoritative, but, said others, the writing would be too uneven to make good reading. Then one day in 1989, in the home of the late Dr. Dan Cunningham of Oxford, England, one of us (JTR) learned that Cunningham himself, along with Piers Nye, a younger Oxford colleague, had studied the life and work of one of our chosen pioneers. Another Oxford colleague, the late Dr. Robert Torrance, had studied the life of yet another. We simply could not ignore their efforts. To try to get the best of both worlds, we chose a compromise: writings by different authors to get the expertise, edited by us to achieve a more even presentation. Since authors rarely appreciate having editors alter their writing, tempers have occasionally flared, perhaps with good reason. Yet the book somehow survived. We are deeply grateful for the patience and graciousness of the authors in allowing our vision for this book to emerge. If it finds an audience, the authors deserve the credit; if it does not, we accept the blame.

Since these are pages from Colorado's colorful history, we have chosen to present first the story of two farm boys whose lives, educations, and careers unfolded almost entirely within Colorado itself. One, George Glover, was one of three students in the first graduating class (1884) of the Colorado Agricultural College, now Colorado State University. The other, Isaac Newsom, was Glover's talented protégé. Although these two men are remembered as educators by their university—and justly so—we show them in a different light, namely, as researchers of heart failure in cattle at high altitude in South Park, Colorado, in 1913. How was it that with almost no resources and many responsibilities they opened a new field of medical research that has important implications for human medicine? And what in their makeup stimulated their students and others to carry on their work? Chapter 1 tells the story.

Preceding the altitude research of Glover and Newsom by two years was the 1911 Anglo-American expedition to Pikes Peak led by John Scott Haldane of Oxford, England. This was the first medical expedition to high altitude in the Western Hemisphere. Furthermore, it laid the foundations for nearly all our understanding of high-altitude acclimatization. Endowed with a complicated personality, Haldane was driven and hardheaded but was also a most compassionate champion of the workingman. Yet, when brilliant scientists have brilliant hunches, on occasion they may be wrong. In Haldane's case, did his error from the Pikes Peak expedition ruin his career? Why does this error continue to haunt his memory even now, decades after his death? Chapter 2 tells the story.

Accompanying Haldane on his 1911 expedition to Colorado was a thirty-nine-year-old woman, Mabel Purefoy FitzGerald, resolute, independent, and adventurous. Faced with the Victorian prohibitions of her gender, which prevented her from entering Oxford University and from working with the men in their research on Pikes Peak, how could she make a lasting scientific contribution and become the only woman researcher featured in these pages? Further, how was she able to overcome Victorian aversions to a single woman going it alone to Colorado's mining camps in wild and high mountains? But she had the last word, as told in chapter 3.

Surely high altitude is a heartfelt stress. In the summer of 1929, when a Johns Hopkins medical student named Arthur Grollman brought Anna Louise, his bride of three years, to the summit of Pikes Peak, he wanted to see how low oxygen affected their hearts. He was surprised by some of his findings and conducted some startling follow-up studies on his return to Baltimore. If one wishes to examine the life of a goal-directed scientist who had scant regard for life's comforts or even his own safety, chapter 4 is certainly a good place to start.

When picturing a dedicated scientist, people usually think of a serious, introverted, quiet individual who plans his experiments and career in advance. But that picture does not fit Bruce Dill, a high-school coach who led a team of Harvard research scientists to Leadville, Colorado, to study human exercise. Maybe in science, as in other walks of life, detailed planning counts less than an honest, inquiring mind, respect and love for mankind, and an ability to lead. Such traits led Dill from humble origins to the presidency of one of the world's premier scientific organizations, the American Physiological Society. Bruce Dill was beloved by all, including us, who had the good fortune to know him, as the reader shall see in chapter 5.

After you have changed the course of your life to help your new boss solve a problem, then how do you feel when, after you have solved it, your boss doesn't believe you and maybe doesn't even care? This was John Lichty's experience in Colorado. In 1947 the problem was to find out why Colorado babies were born so small and had such a high mortality rate. The solution lay in Colorado's altitudes, and it provided clues for small babies born anywhere. The problem Lichty solved was far from trivial, so why was he ignored? The reader must judge in chapter 6.

When Charles Houston, a family doctor in the small town of Aspen, Colorado, rescued a young skier from certain death on a high mountain pass near the Maroon Bells—and then found he had treated a disease that neither he nor any other physician in the United States had ever recognized—it all became a puzzling high adventure. How did he find sober skiers on New Year's Eve 1958 and form a rescue team able to get to 12,000 feet in an impending storm? And what about the victim, Alex Drummond, lying alone in the snow and afraid that death would arrive before the rescuers? The story is told in chapter 7.

Colorado, with the highest average elevation of any state in the United States, has a continuing tradition of rich adventure in medical research. Although we have focused here on those who carried out the researches, no small amount of credit is due to the citizens of Colorado, in Leadville and other high-altitude communities, who have willingly and enthusiastically been the subjects for these research studies. Because of them, Colorado is one of the most important natural high-altitude laboratories for medical research in the world. If this book provides insight into these Colorado pioneers and engenders within the citizens themselves a feeling of adventure and a sense of pride, it will have succeeded.

—JOHN T. REEVES, M.D., AND
ROBERT F. GROVER, M.D., PH.D.

ACKNOWLEDGMENTS

The editors and authors wish to thank those persons, named and un-named, who, by contributing advice, interest, and historical insights or by reading the manuscripts, made this book possible.

For chapter 2, the authors thank the following for substantial and enlightening contributions: Professor Abe Guz, Dr. Brian Lloyd, the late Naomi Mitchison, Professor Denny Mitchison, David O'Connor, Dr. Rosemary Painter, Dr. David Paterson, Dr. Peter Robbins, and the late Dr. Robert Torrance. We thank Professor John Widdicombe for copies of photographs he acquired from Douglas's effects and acknowledge especially the contribution of the late Dr. Dan Cunningham, who was to have been the senior author of this chapter.

For chapter 3, the editors are grateful to Margaret Torrance for her assistance, particularly after her husband's death. We thank Dr. J. M. H. Moll, the editor of the *Journal of Medical Biography*, for permission to use some of the material from Torrance's article in the journal on FitzGerald, and the Bodleian Library for the use of some of the photographs.

For chapter 4 on the Grollmans, the authors are most grateful to Evelyn Grollman of the National Institutes of Health, Baltimore, Maryland, who provided many of the photographs used in this chapter and suggested the title. Thomas Maren gave important information regarding E. K. Marshall, and Harry Fritts provided helpful discussions. The Pioneers Museum in Colorado Springs, particularly Leah Davis-Witherow, and the Johns Hopkins Historical Collection were sources of relevant materials.

For chapter 5 on Dill, the authors are grateful to Dr. J. R. Pappenheimer, Dr. Henry Blackburn, Duane Monk, and Dr. Steven Horvath for their assistance.

For chapter 6 on Lichty, the people of Leadville, Colorado, and the St. Vincent's Hospital medical staff provided the essential cooperation that made the original studies possible and the continuing studies such a pleasure to perform. Juanita Galvan, the late Roger H. Lichty, Dr. Joseph S. Lichty, Dr. Lula Lubchenco, Dr. Rosalind Ting, Dr. Susan Niermeyer, Donald Davids, Bobbi Siegel, Dr. E. Stewart Taylor, and Dr. Stacy Zamudio provided invaluable assistance in the assembly of the historical record, collection of the pertinent documents, and scientific observations. A previous version of this chapter was given as a medical conference at Loma Linda University on February 2, 1990, upon the kind invitation of Dr. Larry Longo.

For chapter 7 on Houston and Drummond, the editors thank J. B. Thomas for his photographs of the Drummond rescue, forwarded by Edward Burlingame. We also thank Barbara Hultgren for the photograph and information on her late husband, and Robert Bates for his comments.

Special thanks are due to those who previewed the manuscript, Gene and Rosann McCullough, Tom Noel, Thomas Schmidt, Robert Shikes, Margaret Torrance, Wiltz Wagner, Elizabeth Weir, and Leah Davis Witherow. Finally we are also grateful for the sponsorship of the Pulmonary Circulation Foundation, which will be the beneficiary of any royalties generated.

CONTRIBUTORS

DAVID BRUCE DILL JR., M.A., geologist, retired

ALEX DRUMMOND, B.S., environmentalist and author

ARTHUR P. GROLLMAN, M.D., professor and chairman, Department of Pharmacology, University of New York Medical School at Stony Brook, New York

ROBERT F. GROVER, M.D., PH.D., professor emeritus of medicine, University of Colorado Health Sciences Center

CHARLES S. HOUSTON, M.D., professor emeritus of medicine, University of Vermont

LORNA GRINDLAY MOORE, PH.D., professor of anthropology, University of Colorado, and professor of medicine, University of Colorado Health Sciences Center

PIERS C. NYE, PH.D., university lecturer, University Laboratory of Physiology, and fellow of Balliol College, Oxford

JOHN T. REEVES, M.D., professor emeritus of medicine, pediatrics, and family medicine, University of Colorado Health Sciences Center

ROBERT W. TORRANCE, M.A., B.SC., B.M., B.CH., university lecturer emeritus, University Laboratory of Physiology, and emeritus fellow of St. John's College, Oxford

ATTITUDES ON ALTITUDE

1
FAILING HEARTS AT HIGH ALTITUDE
"Brisket Disease" in Cattle Teaches Humans a Medical Lesson
Robert F. Grover, M.D., Ph.D.

How could two veterinarians, George Glover and Isaac Newsom, working in isolation on an obscure disease of cattle early in the twentieth century, not only make medical history, but also profoundly affect the careers of young men who never knew them? Robert F. Grover, M.D., Ph.D., tells their story along with his own, for he is one of the young men whose career they influenced. Grover himself had a distinguished career, not only in the study of brisket disease with veterinary colleagues, but also as director of the Cardiopulmonary Research Laboratory at the University of Colorado Health Sciences Center. In 1984 the biennial Grover Conferences on Pulmonary Circulation were established in his honor.

—John T. Reeves

South Park is a broad, shallow valley in the Colorado Rockies, lying in the shadow of Pikes Peak. This ancient lake bed became fertile grassland and was occupied by the Ute Indians until the arrival of the pioneers in the nineteenth century. It appeared to be well suited for grazing livestock, but when ranchers began importing cattle, many died of "brisket disease" (fig. 1.1), whereas the cattle that survived went on to reproduce, and soon stable herds of healthy, acclimatized native cattle were established. These events on this high grassland have had important implications for human medicine, helping physicians better understand lethal heart problems in young children, adolescents, and adults. But at the outset there was no thought of a connection to human medicine; rather it was a problem of economic survival for the cattlemen in South Park.

What accounted for this high mortality among imported cattle? Whereas I have always thought of South Park as a very pleasant huge

1

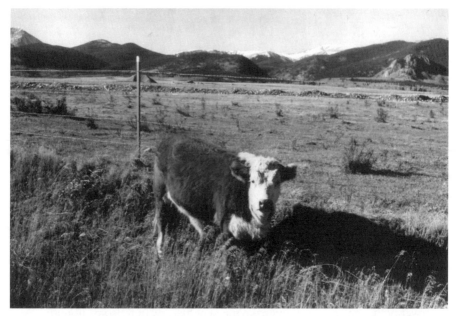

Fig. 1.1. Steer with brisket disease in South Park, Colorado, elevation 10,000 feet. Note swelling of tissues below neck. Peaks in background rise 13,000 to 14,000 feet. Photograph by Robert F. Grover.

meadow, it is in fact at an altitude of 8,000 to 10,000 feet, and the surrounding summer pastures are even higher. As we shall see, it is this high altitude that is the lethal element for some cattle. In medicine, many illnesses bear the name of the physician who first described the condition. For example, Alzheimer's disease is so named for the nineteenth-century German neurologist Alois Alzheimer. By analogy, the unsuspecting person might assume that some early French pathologist such as Jacques Brisket lent his name to brisket disease. Not so. The name "brisket disease" originated with the ranchers themselves and simply implies disease of the brisket of beef, which in fact it is not.

Obviously any condition that results in the loss of many cattle is of major concern to a rancher. Hence in April 1913 two South Park stockmen, Lew W. Robbins and David Collard, advanced one hundred dollars each, a sizable sum in those days. The money was placed at the disposal of the Experiment Station at Colorado Agricultural College (now Colorado State University) in Fort Collins for the study of brisket disease. At the time George H. Glover was the veterinarian at the Experiment Station. He called upon his friend Isaac E. Newsom, a pathologist, and together they proceeded to examine cattle in South Park (fig.

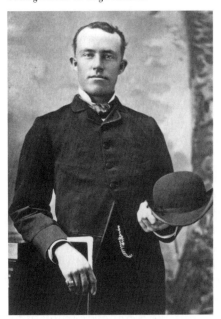 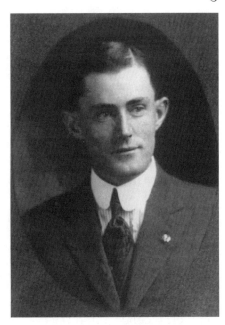

Fig. 1.2. Left, George H. Glover in a student photo; right, Isaac E. Newsom. The two men first established that brisket disease was heart failure caused by exposure to high altitude. Courtesy College of Veterinary Medicine and Biomedical Sciences, Colorado State University, Fort Collins.

1.2). Two years later they published their preliminary survey of brisket disease, with supplemental information in 1917 and detailed case reports in 1918.

Glover and Newsom began their work by interviewing the ranchers. Just how great was the economic impact of brisket disease in Colorado? "During the winter of 1913–1914, one South Park stockman estimates that out of between four and five hundred cattle, he lost thirty calves and ten or twelve older animals. Still another man lost 12 during the winter of 1912–1913. Still another says, after several years' experience, he has lost practically all bulls that he shipped in from low altitude and he figures his loss at about five per cent. . . . While this may seem small, yet in the aggregate it means many thousands of dollars" (Glover and Newsom 1915).

From these interviews they also learned that brisket disease had been known in South Park since 1889 at elevations between 9,000 and 10,000 feet. It had been noticed frequently by the ranchers in North Park at 8,000 feet and near the town of Divide at 9,000 feet, but not at altitudes below 8,000 feet in Colorado's San Luis Valley. Although the disease was usually more frequent in the winter, it also appeared in the summer among cattle pastured at altitudes up to 13,000 feet. Thus right at the outset they suspected a causal role for high altitude. If brisket disease was a disorder of high altitude, perhaps it occurred in other western states, so letters were written to Utah, Wyoming, Montana, Idaho, Nevada, and California. Although veterinarians in these other states replied that they were not familiar with the disease, Glover and Newsom remained confident it would be found at high altitude.

Time proved them to be correct. Three years later they wrote that "the disease is known definitely to exist in Wyoming and New Mexico" (Glover and Newsom 1918), and an extensive report of brisket disease in Utah appeared forty years later (Hecht et al. 1959). Further, we now know that brisket disease is reported to have claimed 90 percent of cattle from Virginia that were shipped to Peru in 1953 and taken to altitudes of 10,800 to 12,200 feet (Hultgren and Spickard 1960).

Glover and Newsom mapped out their plan of attack: "first, to determine whether the disease could be transmitted from one animal to another; second to find the cause; third to make a complete study of its various manifestations; and fourth to find a remedy" (1915). They found the disease was not transmitted to healthy cattle either by exposing them to affected cattle or by injecting them with blood from affected cattle. They ruled against infection because affected cattle had no fever; there was no tenderness or warmth over the brisket; fluids from the animals were not purulent and had no foul odor; and the heart valves were free of vegetations that can be caused by colonies of bacteria. They ruled out the problem of the feed, or some infectious agent in it, because hay shipped from North and South Park to lower altitudes did not cause the disease. From these studies they concluded that brisket disease was not "transmissible or even infectious."

What they found was heart failure, "a swelling of the loose tissues under the jaw and a swelling of the loose tissues of the brisket. . . . Gradually the two merge into each other as the whole under part of the neck becomes *dropsical* . . . [and] may become enormous in size" (italics mine). The swelling was a collection of tissue fluid that we call edema of heart failure but that in those days was called "dropsy," a term that appears in the subtitle to their article (Glover and Newsom 1915). As the heart fails to pump blood forward to the tissues, the pulse becomes weak, and as blood backs up, the veins, including those in the neck, become engorged. Glover and Newsom duly noted the weak pulse and the distended neck veins. The cattle had other signs of failure. They were short of breath, and only slight exertion raised the heart rate to 120 beats per minute, which is three times the normal resting rate in cattle. (The human analogy would be if simply walking across the room caused a heart rate of 180.) Continued exertion often caused death in these brisket-disease cattle.

When they examined cattle that had died, they found large and flabby hearts. The blood that had backed up from the heart into the veins and capillaries had caused the liver to become swollen with blood (Glover and Newsom 1918). Because pressure in the capillaries had caused them to leak, edema fluid accumulated in many tissues, including the intestines, which explained the profuse diarrhea—known to ranchers as "scours"—a prominent feature of brisket disease. Many liters of edema fluid found their way into the abdominal and chest cavities, which are normally nearly dry. These were all findings of heart failure.

Heart failure in cattle is similar to that in humans, except that in cattle the legs are spared. In humans with congestive heart failure, the effect of gravity causes edema fluid to collect first in the dependent parts of the body, the feet, ankles, and legs. In four-legged animals, heart-failure fluid likewise accumulates in the dependent parts of the body, but not in the legs, because the tight ligaments and sheaths are strong enough to prevent accumulation. Rather, the fluid accumulates in the next most dependent portions of the body—under the loose skin of the chest and neck. Of course there is nothing wrong with the muscles beneath the skin, the so-called brisket (from which we make corned beef), so "brisket disease" is really a misnomer. Glover and Newsom wrote: "Lancing the swollen brisket and placing various medicaments within can do no good and is to be considered barbarous. It is in line with slitting the tail and putting in salt and pepper, and like the latter practice it should be eliminated as soon as possible" (Glover and Newsom 1915).

If, as Glover and Newsom suspected, high altitude was the cause of the heart failure, then the failure should disappear when the animals were sent lower. So in November of 1913 they shipped a steer with brisket disease from 9,500 feet in Jefferson, Colorado, in South Park to Denver at 5,280 feet. Not only did the swollen brisket and diarrhea completely disappear in two weeks, but the animal recovered its vigor and began to fatten normally. They reported: "Altogether there have been six cases shipped from a high altitude (9,500 to 11,000 feet) to a lower one (5,000 to 5,280) and in each case prompt recovery followed. In no case was any medicinal treatment given." From all this, Glover and Newsom were convinced that altitude had caused heart failure. Thus, they subtitled their report "Dropsy of High Altitude."

In at least one other respect, namely, genetics, Glover and Newsom were well ahead of their time: "Calves sired by bulls from low altitudes are more likely to be affected than those sired by native bulls. . . . The remedy lies not in drugs, but in breeding a hardier strain of cattle." They also anticipated the genetic concept of "individual variability" by recognizing that not all cattle brought to high altitude would develop brisket disease. But those that do "would undoubtedly give rise to a certain number of offspring whose hearts would be insufficient to meet the vigorous conditions. . . . It [brisket disease] is brought about by exertion before acclimatization at high altitudes, or in the case of calves, inherited cardiac weakness" (Glover and Newsom 1915). Remarkably, the concept that susceptibility to brisket disease is inherited but varies markedly from one individual to the next was proven correct (Cruz et al. 1980; Will et al. 1975) and even extended to other species, including humans (Grover et al. 1963b), but only many years later.

Glover and Newsom had two pieces of the brisket-disease puzzle—reduced oxygen at altitude and heart failure (1917). Lacking a third piece, that low oxygen (hypoxia) causes the small lung arteries to constrict, they connected the two they had and speculated that low oxygen had directly caused the heart to fail. That the understanding of hypoxia in 1915 was less than it is today should not detract from their truly remarkable piece of work. Not until 1946, thirty years later, did two Scandinavian investigators, von Euler and Liljestrand, demonstrate in cats that breathing a hypoxic gas for a few minutes slightly raised the pressure in the pulmonary artery, thereby increasing slightly the work of the right ventricle of the heart. They speculated that the low oxygen had caused the small pulmonary arteries to constrict. It was yet another ten years before researchers in Colorado and Utah (Alexander and Jensen 1959; Alexander et al. 1960; Hecht et al. 1959) learned that chronic hypoxia was far more powerful than acute hypoxia in narrowing small lung arteries. Certainly back in 1915 there was no way Glover and Newsom could have known that low oxygen had so narrowed these small arteries as to obstruct blood flow through the lungs and thus cause the heart to fail.

Why, one wonders, would nature want low oxygen to constrict lung arteries? Surely over the eons of time, such a mechanism has not evolved in order simply to sicken cattle at high altitude. Nature's "purpose" seems to be more elegant, extending perhaps even to the preservation of cattle and other mammalian species by using the oxygen level to control the lung arteries in the unborn and newborn. While the fetus is in the womb, the useless lungs have a very low oxygen level, which constricts their arteries so that they receive little blood flow and more flow is available to receive oxygen in the placenta. With the onset of breathing at birth, the high oxygen levels in the air entering the lungs now help dilate lung arteries, so that a large blood flow can now receive oxygen in the lungs. In providing for an oxygen supply to the unborn and newborn, nature's strategy is brilliant: low oxygen constricts fetal lung arteries when the lung is not needed, and after birth high oxygen in the air dilates lung arteries when the lung becomes essential. Although this control of the small lung arteries by oxygen is essential for survival before birth and immediately afterward, it persists throughout life, but gets weaker with age.

If low oxygen constricts lung arteries more strongly in the young than in the old, then young calves should be more susceptible than adults to heart failure at altitude. In fact, Glover and Newsom realized that young calves were very susceptible to brisket disease, "even calves as young as one month often showing well marked symptoms" (1917). And in the seventeen cases reported in detail (Glover and Newsom 1918) only one was older than three years and twelve were age one year or less, the youngest being only six weeks old. Some years later investigators confirmed the propensity of brisket disease to strike the young (Hecht et al. 1959; Pierson and Jensen 1956). In 1915 Glover and Newsom had no way of knowing about the lung circulation of the fetus and newborn, but their report presages an important subsequent concept, namely, the lung circulation in the very young has heightened susceptibility to hypoxia. Today, when babies are born at high altitude, they routinely receive oxygen, and so do newborn babies at any altitude, when they have life-threatening constriction of lung arteries.

With these classic studies showing that brisket disease was heart failure due to low oxygen at high altitude, that it had a genetic component, that susceptibility varied among animals, and that the young were often afflicted, Glover and Newsom joined that select group of scientists we now recognize as pioneers in high-altitude research in Colorado. As with several other pioneers included in this volume, in spite of the landmark nature of their work on brisket disease, their four papers from 1915 to 1918 constituted their only excursion into high-altitude research. Today Glover and Newsom are remembered at Colorado State University for their many contributions in developing the institution itself, but their pioneering work on brisket disease is rarely mentioned.

Just who were these pioneers, Glover and Newsom? Both had humble beginnings as farm boys. George Henry Glover was born in Iowa in 1864. When he was seven, his family moved to Colorado to continue farming near Longmont. At age sixteen and extremely shy, Glover entered the newly opened agricultural college in nearby Fort Collins after first securing a janitorial job to cover expenses. Fortunately on arriving he met President Edwards. When Glover turned out to be too shy to sign up for classes, Edwards, wondering what had happened to the boy, went to his room and personally led him to register (Hansen 1977). As a student Glover was required to deliver a "public oration" once each term, a traumatic experience he vividly recalled: "I became nervous, lost all desire for food and was sure I could perceive the symptoms of nervous prostration. I walked the campus without thought of direction and finally, as I came to the railroad I stopped, looked longingly toward home and was suddenly overcome by an irresistible impulse. When I next became conscious of my actions, I was headed south for Longmont . . . and I never stopped until I got there" (McGuire and Hansen 1983).

Somehow his college career did survive, and in 1884 Glover and two other intrepid individuals constituted the first class to graduate from the new Colorado Agricultural College. But who would have predicted that during the next twenty-five years George Glover would have selected a career of teaching, that is, giving "public orations" before the students, or that he would have attained national prominence as president of the American Veterinary Medical Association?

Apparently at least one faculty member recognized that this student had talent: "On commencement day he [Glover] was in his dormitory room practicing his senior oration . . . when he was interrupted by a knock at the door. Expecting another student, Glover shouted out an abusive epithet, and became embarrassed when the dignified Professor Lawrence walked in. Lawrence said that he had learned of his [Glover's] interest in pursuing graduate work in veterinary medicine at Iowa. . . . He then offered to lend the boy money for this purpose with no collateral or interest. At first Glover was too overwhelmed to respond. 'Well,' the professor asked, 'will you do it?' 'Will a duck swim?' answered the boy" (Hansen 1977).

Following graduation and with the help of the loan, he went on to study veterinary medicine at Iowa State Agricultural College, obtaining his degree in veterinary medicine one year later in 1885. He then returned to Colorado, where he became state inspector for cattle herds in Colorado and also Montana. Because of an epidemic of "Texas fever" in the herds in 1886, he is reported as having examined 242,000 head of cattle in that single year (Peake 1937). In 1901, at the age of thirty-seven, he was appointed head of the newly established Department of Veterinary Science at Colorado Agricultural College (fig. 1.3).

Glover believed strongly that the veterinary faculty had an obligation to assist the farmers and ranchers of Colorado and that this service could best be provided through extension activity, as well as research involving animal maladies. Glover's own research was on poisonous plants that accounted for livestock losses amounting to two million dol-

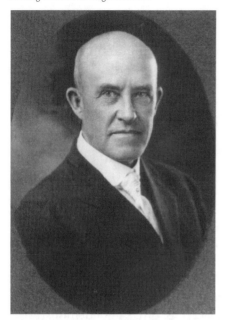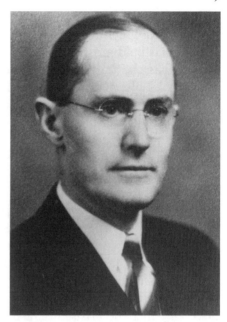

Fig. 1.3. Left, George H. Glover, first dean of the College of Veterinary Medicine; right, Isaac E. Newsom, who succeeded Glover as dean. Courtesy College of Veterinary Medicine and Biomedical Sciences, Colorado State University, Fort Collins.

lars in a single year. In recognition of this valuable work he was selected to fill the position of Experiment Station veterinarian in 1904.

Finding that the demands for veterinary services were more than a single department could meet, Glover saw the need for a full-fledged School of Veterinary Medicine in Colorado; there were fewer than twenty in the country and only four were state supported. But he had not been able to convince the board of the Colorado Agricultural College. However, he hit upon a plan after he had examined the college dairy herd and had found several cows that might be infected with tuberculosis. "He invited the board members and other dignitaries to witness the slaughter of some extremely valuable livestock. Glover had some doubts, for the diagnosis was not foolproof. . . . Glancing at the prominent visitors, he took a deep breath and sank his knife into a suspect cow. Quickly, . . . he discovered the lungs and glands to be rotten with the disease. Confident of the demonstration's success, Glover could not resist a flamboyant touch. Carefully removing a nodule in the udder, he held it for his audience to see, then sliced the abnormal growth, which burst out with a sickening mixture of milk and pus. . . . 'That,' said Glover, 'is what you've been selling people for milk' " (Hansen

1977). The demonstration showed that Glover had gotten over much of his timidity, which like the wave in his hair proved to be transient, for Glover was bald most of his life. Considering that in those years tuberculosis was the leading cause of death in humans, the demonstration succeeded beyond his imagination, for it began the drive for milk and meat inspection laws, first in Fort Collins and then throughout Colorado. Not only did tuberculosis begin to decline, but also, in 1907, the college board approved a full course of study leading to the Doctor of Veterinary Science Degree.

However, the problems were far from over. The fledgling program failed to receive accreditation by the United States Department of Agriculture because the faculty was perceived as being undermanned and insufficiently qualified. No wonder. Glover's staff was composed only of himself and two "associate professors," Isaac E. Newsom and Harry E. Kingman Sr., both of whom Glover had trained as student assistants. It was a crisis for veterinary education in Colorado. In order to understand better the character of these men, I wanted to know the details of how they met the crisis, because character is often best demonstrated in adversity. Glover, Newsom, and Kingman, of course, were not living, but I was able to find and interview the son of one of them, Harry E. Kingman Jr.

He recalled the crisis this way:

> The accreditation board came out here and said, your faculty isn't good enough. So dad and Newsom got together and they both went to Kansas City; in fact, the two families lived in the same apartment house close together. It took about six or seven months at Kansas City Veterinary College, and then after that Newsom went to San Francisco to one of the private veterinary schools out there. Dad went to Chicago to McKillips, where they were teaching pretty much horse practice because Chicago was a booming horse-drawn town. This time away from Fort Collins greatly broadened their experience. . . .
> During their absence Benjamin Kaupp and Clarence Barnes, two veterinarians in private practice around Fort Collins, came out and filled in for them. Also, Dr. Carrie, a physician in town, got a bunch of doctors to sign up for classes to raise the number of students to keep the school open.

In this manner, with Glover at the helm, and with the remarkable efforts of Newsom and Kingman, the school struggled through many very difficult months, culminating in 1909 with the attainment of full accreditation together with congratulations from the committee of the U.S. Department of Agriculture. In a very real sense, then, the survival and subsequent success of the veterinary school may be credited largely to the determination, dedication, and personal sacrifice of three men, George Glover, Isaac Newsom, and Harry Kingman Sr.

But even such dedication was not enough. As Harry Kingman Jr. explained, "Everybody on the faculty had to have outside income of some sort or they didn't survive. The salaries were absolutely poor. Glover did city meat inspections. Newsom was the pathologist and had the contract with the hospital General Valley or whatever it was called at that time. He did all the tissue work for the hospital and along with it bacteriology for the public health department. . . . Dad had a private practice . . . and he was on ambulatory call as well as working at the hospital. He had to buy his own drugs and his own gasoline and take kids [students] out on calls, for which he charged them. He had to collect his own bills. Every Saturday and Sunday he would deliver calves at the only Hereford ranch, work for two days, and come back to teach on Monday." Academic life at the beginning of the twentieth century was not easy; it was one of uncertainty and even poverty. These dedicated men did whatever it took in pursuit of their vision.

Their efforts paid off. Once firmly established, the Department of Veterinary Medicine flourished under Glover's direction. Meanwhile, Glover continued his major responsibility as veterinarian for the Experiment Station, which he saw as an important vehicle for responding to the health needs of the state. His effective use of the Station essentially eliminated tuberculosis in Colorado's dairy herds by 1909. Also, he used the station to educate ranchers about weeds poisonous to livestock, thereby controlling this problem. In 1912 hog growers in the San Luis Valley had turned to the Station for assistance with what proved to be an epidemic of hog cholera; Glover brought this under control. Thus it was natural for him to respond in 1913, when cattlemen in South Park called upon the Station for help with the problem of brisket disease.

With their successes in brisket disease, why did Glover and Newsom never return to the problem? Being practical men, perhaps they saw other problems needing attention; for Glover, plants that poisoned livestock, and for Newsom, feedlot diseases of sheep. The agitation by cattlemen must have subsided. And why not? The investment of one hundred dollars each by Robbins and Collard had paid off handsomely. Cattlemen now knew that brisket disease was from altitude; the affected animals need not die, for they could be shipped lower and there fatten for market; and judicious breeding could mainly prevent the problem. The U.S. National Institutes of Health, which currently spends billions yearly for heart and lung research, could easily be envious of such a return on research dollars.

Even with all their duties, both Glover and Newsom taught classes. Wanting to know more about their personalities, I sought persons who had been their students. How one faces adversity may define character, but how one faces the classroom is a window on personality. I was able to locate and interview four of their former students, John Thimmig, Bill Harrison, Harry Kingman Jr., and Ken Smith. Ken's wife, Nina, provided additional insights.

Thimmig smiled and commented: "I can remember about the second lecture that we had with Glover; he was standing in front with his eyes closed. You knew he wasn't asleep because he was talking. He said, 'This is a course in jurisprudence, that is, medical law. True, we do have a textbook. You fellows can read that textbook just as well as I can, but it isn't very often that you get a chance to listen to an old fellow like me.' We would have class once a week. Philosophy, anything that came to his mind. He made his lectures enjoyable because of his homespun philosophy. He would weave new threads into an old coat. He was really good."

Harrison recalled: "Glover didn't speak rapidly. He spoke slow but so interesting that you followed him. It was easy to follow his line of thinking. A wonderful lecturer. I thought his ability to lecture and to keep your attention was much better than a person who would rattle it off very rapidly and expect you to be taking notes along with everything else. About closing his eyes, I think he was visualizing his notes."

Or could this habit have been a remnant of his youthful timidity? As we have seen, Glover overcame many difficulties in his career, including his shyness in public, but perhaps not completely.

Kingman chuckled, "I had a little yellow dog named Hiney who went through school with me. Glover would be teaching, and we would hear a scratch at the door. Glover would look knowingly at me. Then slowly he would go over and open the door. Hiney would come in and lie down at my feet. . . . Glover would then resume his posture, eyes closed once more. If his back itched, he would get up against the corner of the door frame and work at it. Eyes still closed. Glover never quit on time, and when the bell would ring, Hiney would get up and go over and scratch on the door. Glover would then go over and open the door and excuse class. There would be days when . . . Glover would start reminiscing and . . . use up the whole hour, . . . eyes closed . . . until Hiney would scratch at the door. . . . When he kept his eyes closed, he couldn't see what was happening in the room . . . ; if some walked out, he wouldn't even miss them."

In these interviews, my presence and my tape recorder were soon forgotten as these aging scholars recalled their student days fully sixty-five years earlier. The details of their recall and their laughter, which brought tears and sometimes even inhibited speech, were proof positive that they enormously enjoyed the veterinary medicine taught in those early days. And what a fascinating picture of the atmosphere within the classroom, respect mixed with affection, a closeness difficult to imagine today.

———•———

Isaac Ernest Newsom, nearly twenty years younger than Glover, was born in Colorado City, Texas, in 1883, and he too grew up on a farm in Colorado near Parker. The two men nicely complemented each other. Glover's strengths lay in his vision, administration, assembling a talented staff, and public relations. As a testimony of his ability to judge character, he recruited Newsom in 1900 to become an undergraduate student at the College. Newsom's strength lay in a serious, lifelong dedication to intellectual pursuits. As a student, he arrived at his first class having memorized much of the required text. Glover realized that this young man, who craved knowledge and was a voracious reader, also had academic potential. Immediately on Newsom's graduation in 1904 Glover appointed him to the faculty.

Glover was not disappointed in his younger colleague. Newsom's ability to recognize problems, formulate solutions, and conduct research is apparent in the reports on brisket disease (Glover and Newsom 1915, 1917, 1918; Newsom 1915). Obviously he had reviewed the scant existing literature dealing with the effects of altitude on the human heart, and he was familiar with Haldane's papers (see chap. 2). Then, with his exceptional talent for analysis, it is likely Newsom considered how altitude might affect oxygen supply to heart muscle. Almost certainly, the logical plan of attack on the brisket-disease problem (Glover and Newsom 1915) was the result of Newsom's touch. He was inherently a research scientist.

Perhaps nowhere was the personality difference between Glover and Newsom seen more clearly than in the classroom, as attested by the former students of both men. Harrison described Newsom this way: "The knot on Newsom's tie was always properly tied. He was immaculate in his approach to anything he did, whether it was his notes, his lecture, his dress, or anything. He was simply immaculate. Everyone respected and loved him. From the moment he stepped in front of the class you knew that you were dealing with an intellectual. We were blessed with a faculty person like Newsom. And he loved rituals. Masonic Order. I don't know what he did in Masonry, but he was a big wheel."

Thimmig added, "Newsom was wonderful to me. If you just walked into his class and he was standing up in front, you would think this is a stern individual. But he was warmhearted."

Harrison agreed. "I think that was because he didn't smile a lot. He kept his facial expressions the same all the time. So you would have that impression that he was a stern individual. He certainly wasn't. The minute you got to know him he was warm. Although he spoke in a kind of monotone, he had ways of lecturing that were actually very expressive, and you didn't miss a word of his lectures. I had him for part of a class, diseases of sheep and poultry. He managed to call it 'Breeding and Feeding the Bucks and Ducks.'"

Along with his dry sense of humor he energized his students by introducing them to his innovative research into sheep losses in feedlots, forage poisoning of horses, contagious abortion, and of course brisket disease in cattle. His material was new, exciting, and practical. Dignified and gentlemanly, he had the universal respect and confidence of students and faculty alike.

Kingman brought out a yellowed publication dated 1929 and turned to an article by Newsom that illustrates his candor. The opening paragraph reads: "It would seem that the literature on coccidiosis in cattle is already so voluminous as to require no addition from me. The only excuse therefore, for this article is the request of the editor who seemingly wanted a summary of present information put into a condensed form where it might be available without an exhaustive search of the literature." Many a scientist asked to write a review article might have similar sentiments, but how many would have the courage to express them so candidly in print?

Such honesty and a serious, dignified mien apparently hid from view a rather boisterous spirit, as illustrated by two student pranks. It seems that Newsom was a member of one of the school's two oratorical societies. During a competition, when a member of the opposition rose to speak, a banner dropped down from above, suddenly shutting the speaker off from the audience. Newsom's role in the prank and the riot that followed is not clear, but his name was prominent when the event was recalled (Hansen 1977).

Nina Smith added this anecdote of a second prank: "The president's house was the original part of Old Main . . . [and] every time there was a fire alarm the president would come racing down the stairs to check it out. To hear Newsom tell it, he and a bunch of the students got together and covered the banister with 'moist corral dust'; he couldn't bring him-

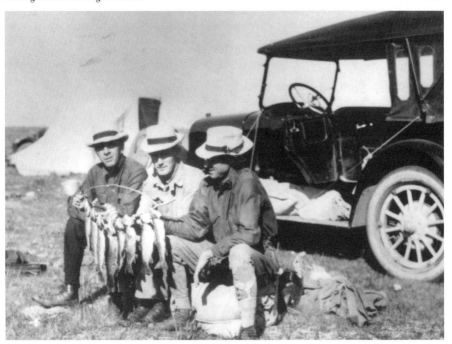

Fig. 1.4. "Ike" Newsom (center) with two of his fishing buddies, Dick Bourne (left) and Harry Kingman Sr. (right), ca 1925. Courtesy of Harry Kingman Jr.

self to use the word 'manure.' Then they turned in a false alarm, and as the president came down [the stairs] he was practically covered from head to foot with the moist corral dust."

What a great story! Newsom, who was so fastidious about his own appearance, must have been quite amazed to see the president of the university covered with manure. That Newsom could tell this story on himself and laugh at his own role in the episode speaks volumes about his sense of humor, which undoubtedly contributed to his ability to get on with people. His classroom demeanor belied the informal side of his personality, easily seen, for example, on relaxed fishing trips with his colleagues (fig. 1.4).

Though opposites in personality, Glover and Newsom remained close friends and fully dedicated to the educational program in veterinary science throughout their careers. In 1934, twenty-seven years after establishing the Department of Veterinary Science, Glover became the first dean of the School of Veterinary Medicine. In 1918 Newsom had been appointed head of the newly organized pathology department, and in 1934 he succeeded Glover as the second dean of veterinary

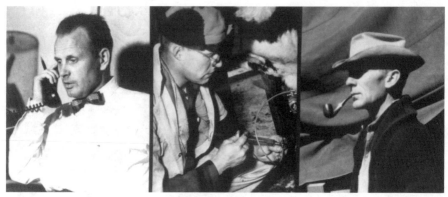

Fig. 1.5. Left, *Rue Jensen, who became dean of the College of Veterinary Medicine in 1957. He nurtured the "golden age of research" at Colorado State University and revived the interest in brisket disease. Archibald F. Alexander (center), a graduate student under Rue Jensen, together with Donald H. Will (right), a circulatory physiologist, continued the study of brisket disease. Photograph of Jensen Courtesy of College of Veterinary Medicine and Biomedical Sciences, Colorado State University, Fort Collins. Photographs of Alexander and Will by Robert F. Grover.*

medicine (fig. 1.3), a post that he held until 1948 when he became president of the college, then renamed Colorado A&M.

Harry Kingman Sr., the third member of the original triumvirate of the fledgling Department of Veterinary Science in 1909, became the first head of the Department of Surgery and Clinics in 1934 and remained with the school as a clinical professor until his retirement. All three, Glover, Newsom, and Kingman, lived into their eighties and witnessed the growth and development of what is now Colorado State University's College of Veterinary Medicine and Biomedical Sciences, one of the finest in the country for both teaching and research. The building of an outstanding educational institution—this, then, is their legacy.

Continuing the Work in Brisket Disease

And what of the brief excursion by Glover and Newsom into the subject of brisket disease eighty years ago? Following their fourth publication in 1918, nothing appeared in the literature for many years. As Newsom continued to lecture about brisket disease, one of his students, Rue Jensen, became the crucial link for continuing the research in Colorado (fig. 1.5). As Jensen said to me, "I credit Newsom for my belief in the theory of hypoxia, and I credit the fascinating [brisket] disease itself for my strong and endless interest in it." Jensen joined the faculty

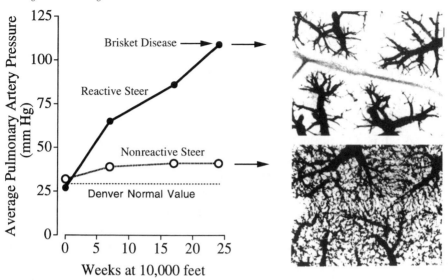

Fig. 1.6. Left, *examples of pulmonary artery pressures in two of ten steers from a Kansas herd at 3,600 feet altitude that were taken to South Park, Colorado, at 10,000 feet, and studied serially over twenty-five weeks. One steer was very reactive to high altitude, had a large increase in pressure, and actually developed heart failure (brisket disease). In contrast another steer was nonreactive to altitude and had only a minimal elevation of pressure. These two steers demonstrate the variability in response among individuals exposed to the same stimulus.*

At postmortem the lungs of these two steers were injected with radio-opaque barium sulfate to visualize their pulmonary arteries. When the X-rays of these lungs were magnified (right), the small arterial branches were seen to be filled in the nonreactive lung (lower right). In contrast the small vessels appear to be "pruned" from the arterial tree of the reactive steer (upper right), i.e., they were so narrowed that they could not be filled with the barium. Reprinted, by permission, from Karger.

following graduation in 1942 and rose rapidly to the rank of full professor in 1948. His wartime appointment in 1943 included responsibility for all anatomical pathology, including teaching, autopsies, and research. By 1945 he had examined hundreds of hearts from cattle, including those with brisket disease.

Jensen found that the right ventricle was dilated and thickened in brisket disease, and not the whole heart as implied by Glover and Newsom. In his 1952 article, "Right Heart Failure," he postulated that the back-up of blood behind the failing right ventricle raised the blood pressure, returning blood to the heart and giving rise to the distention of the neck veins. By 1956 he and Pierson had established that brisket disease occurred with greater frequency in the winter than the summer months, but with equal frequency in males and females. They postulated that "atmospheric hypoxia causes pulmonary changes which lead to increased resistance to circulation through the lungs and failure of the right ventricle," but they weren't sure what those pulmonary changes were.

So what was the nature of this problem in the lung circulation? A substantial research effort was needed. In such a circumstance there is nothing better than the assistance of a bright, energetic young person, and a young graduate student in pathology, Archibald Alexander, arrived to help (fig. 1.5). Working together from 1956 on, Alexander and Jensen found from autopsy studies that high altitude increased the weight of the right ventricle even in healthy cattle, but not nearly as much as in brisket disease (Alexander and Jensen 1959). They found that brisket disease was caused neither by blood clots blocking the lung arteries or, as suggested by human data from Peru (Hurtado et al. 1956; Monge-M. 1928), by excessive production of red blood cells, which make the blood viscous and hard to pump. As useful as these postmortem studies were, heart catheterizations in living cattle were needed to learn what had gone wrong with the lung circulation.

In 1953 and 1954 Jensen had done heart catheterizations in living brisket-disease cattle and had found elevated right-heart pressures, but the records had been lost.[1] To repeat the studies, Jensen then recruited a young veterinarian, Donald Will, who was a circulatory physiologist (fig. 1.5). In early 1957 Jack Reeves and I met Jensen, Alexander, and Will in a frigid barn at 10,000 feet in South Park, Colorado, while they were performing these heart catheterizations in brisket-disease cattle. Since Reeves and I were doing human-heart catheterizations in Denver at the time, we proposed to pool resources from our two institutions and work together, and this proposal was accepted. We now had an expanded team, and Alexander was its captain.

Of course we discussed what might be wrong with the lung that caused the right ventricle to fail in the brisket-disease cattle at high altitude. In 1957 we knew that when mammals breathed low-oxygen mixtures for a few minutes, the pressure in the lung arteries rose (Motley et al. 1947; Von Euler and Liljestrand 1946), but the effect of living for months or years in a low-oxygen environment while residing at high altitude was not known. Possibly a long exposure to low oxygen would raise pressure in the lung arteries much more than a short exposure. To test this idea we brought cattle from low altitude to 10,000 feet in South Park and found they developed markedly elevated pressures in their pulmonary arteries (fig. 1.6), and some cattle even developed brisket disease (Alexander et al. 1960). About this time we learned that an outstanding group at the University of Utah, led by a physician, Hans Hecht, was also doing heart catheterization studies in cattle with brisket disease (Hecht et al. 1959). In 1960 Hecht invited us to a conference in Utah, where we all presented our findings and found that the results in Colorado and in Utah agreed. Thus there was no question that residence at high altitude caused severe pulmonary hypertension, which, in some cattle, led to right-heart failure and even death.

Charles S. Houston, M.D.—of whom more in chapter 7—was a general medical practitioner in Aspen, had attended Hecht's conference in Salt Lake City, and on his return home found how fragile life was for brisket-disease cattle.

> My recollection is that Hans Hecht's meeting was about brisket disease, because I went back to Aspen so puffed up with new knowledge that I soon had another experience: A rancher friend some 20 miles from Aspen called me to ask if I knew anything about brisket disease. (I saw a good many animals with various problems, since the only veterinarian was some distance away.) I said, "Of course I do and I'll be right there." I took my black bag and my electrocardiograph machine, went to the ranch, examined the sorry looking young bull and told the ranch hand to help me attach the electrocardiograph leads. (I was going to do this right!) The bull struggled but was thrown; the leads attached; I only got a straight line. After a long silence, the ranch hand said, "Doc, I think yore patient's daid." And so he was. My rancher friend did not hold against me the death of a $9,000 animal, but for a year or so afterward, whenever I suggested I do an electrocardiogram on a patient, he would hesitate, "Doc, I don't know. I heard what happened to Wirk Cook's bull." (Houston 1999)

When Hecht moved from Utah to Chicago, work on brisket disease effectively ceased in Utah, but the work in Colorado continued.

Alexander launched a very concerted attack on the lung circulation of these cattle. After the lungs were removed from affected animals, they were studied by a special X-ray technique, which showed that the small lung arteries were markedly narrowed, or even blocked (fig. 1.6). When the small lung arteries were examined under the microscope, their walls were greatly thickened (Alexander and Jensen 1963), as if severe, sustained contraction of these arteries had caused the muscle in their walls to thicken and strengthen. Clearly, the blood was forced to flow through very narrow channels, and the force had to come from the right ventricle, which must pump at higher pressure. But when the pressure required became too high, the right ventricle failed. Thus, from both Colorado and Utah, the picture was now clear: many months of low oxygen at high altitude caused constricted lung arteries to obstruct blood flow, leading to brisket disease.

From these early studies in Colorado an alliance was begun that continues to the present day between the School of Veterinary Medicine in Fort Collins and the School of Medicine in Denver. Among the long series of joint projects that have followed, Glover and Newsom would surely be pleased with the confirmation that brisket disease has a heritable component that can be minimized by careful breeding (Cruz et al. 1980; Grover et al. 1963a; Will et al. 1962, 1975).

Did I want to apply the lessons learned to humans? You bet! And so began my personal medical odyssey at high altitude. It was a simple question. If cattle living at high altitude have elevated pulmonary arterial pressures, do people too? I decided to start in North America's highest community, Leadville, Colorado, at 10,152 feet. The year was 1961, about four years after John Lichty had finished his research on low birth weights in Leadville babies (chap. 6). No medical research had been done there since, and none on the lung circulation of adults had ever been done there. Some of my colleagues in Denver assured me there was no problem to be studied and the research would turn up nothing. But the findings in cattle had been so striking that I had to see for myself.

We began with a medical survey consisting of a physical examination, electrocardiogram, and chest X-ray of the students in the Leadville High School (Pryor et al. 1965). It would be difficult to get permission to do this today, and certainly the chest X-rays would not be allowed because of radiation exposure. But in 1961 it was not only possible, but there was such enthusiastic support in Leadville that we examined the entire high-school population—all 508 students.

Sure enough, we found thirty-one students (high-risk group) who almost certainly had elevated pressures in their lung arteries, and in some we worried that the right ventricle of the heart was affected. The only way to be sure was to do a heart catheterization. But was it ethical to submit apparently healthy young men and women to an invasive procedure involving radiation from fluoroscopy? In most cases today the answer would be no. Nowadays one can use echocardiograms and assess the right-ventricle and lung-artery pressure noninvasively, but in 1961 this was not possible. Also in those years there were no human-research committees to provide guidelines and advice. So these issues were discussed with the local physicians, the school authorities, and the parents. In the end, it was decided that the findings were abnormal enough that we should ask the students at greatest risk if they would

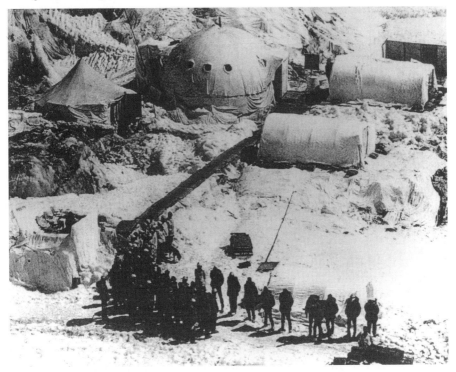

Fig. 1.7. *Military base on a frigid glacier at nearly 20,000 feet on the contested border between India and Pakistan. Under these extreme conditions some soldiers develop "human brisket disease." Reprinted, by permission, from* Time Magazine, *July 31, 1989.*

submit to heart catheterization. Furthermore, on the grounds that our preliminary screening methods were not very precise and that nearly all of the students had some findings that were not normal by low-altitude standards, we should also approach some of the other students, those considered to be at low risk.

Of the thirty-one students in the high-risk group, the first sixteen we approached all readily agreed to have catheterization, and of those in the low-risk group, the first twelve agreed. Why did they agree so readily? They knew that the catheterization procedure was uncomfortable, that it took more than an hour, and that, using local anesthetic, a vein and an artery in one arm had to be surgically exposed. However, as time passed we began to realize that Leadville citizens had long had nagging concerns that the altitude was not entirely benign, and they were delighted that it finally would be looked into.

To see how living at 10,150 feet had affected these young people, the studies should be done in Leadville and not nearly a mile lower in Denver. Leadville's new St. Vincent's Hospital had been recently built, and in the basement the X-ray department had a fluoroscope; there was also some unused space nearby. Heart catheterization was a far simpler matter then than now, but even then it involved a good deal more than a fluoroscope and a spare room. We needed to transport to Leadville everything needed for heart catheterization: sterile drapes and instruments, catheters, monitors, pressure recorders, blood gas analyzers, a bicycle adapted for reclining subjects, high pressure tanks containing oxygen-rich and oxygen-poor air, blood gas analyzers—everything except the fluoroscope. That meant loading an entire laboratory into the back of a truck and crossing the Continental Divide twice—Loveland Pass at 12,000 feet and Fremont Pass at 11,300 feet. With more enthusiasm than good sense, we selected midwinter as the time to start. But we survived the trips and the students survived the catheterizations—all without incident (Grover 1994).

Nearly all the students in Leadville had elevated pressures in their lung arteries. All of the sixteen students at high risk had elevated pressures in their lung arteries, and only one was near the normal Denver value. Eleven of the twelve students at low risk also had elevated lung arterial pressures, though none had pressures that were alarmingly high. As was true in cattle, so in the students, long residence at high altitude had raised the pulmonary arterial pressure in nearly every one, but the amount of the elevation varied greatly from one student to another.

Among the sixteen students considered to be at high risk was a young woman who subsequently required our attention. Like all the other students in the heart catheterization study she felt perfectly well; in fact, she was an outstanding skier at Leadville High School. But we had found that the pressure in her pulmonary artery at rest was three times the normal one and that it more than doubled during mild exercise. These pressures were alarmingly high for they were in the range of values known to be potentially lethal. We and her own physician urged her to leave Leadville and move to a lower altitude. She did move, and after a few months near sea level a repeat heart catheterization showed her pressures at rest and during exercise were normal. She later married, but when she visited Leadville for only a few months, the pressures in her lung arteries shot up again. To have the prospect of a normal life it was necessary for her to return permanently to sea level. Apparently there are some humans who, like some cattle, are susceptible and develop very high pulmonary arterial pressure at high altitude in Colorado. Nature sometimes determines that cattle are the professors and we, the human researchers, are the students. Our current concept that living at high altitude can cause life-threatening pulmonary hypertension has its roots in veterinary medical research done in 1913, nearly fifty years before these human studies in Leadville.

Brisket disease is, by definition, heart failure developing in some cattle after weeks or months of exposure to high altitude. In humans, residence at altitude raises pulmonary arterial pressure, but can it also cause heart failure? The answer is probably yes. In one setting soldiers were stationed in India on the frigid Saichen glacier for over ten weeks at a time at 20,000 feet or even above (fig. 1.7). Even though pressures in the lung arteries have not been measured at that great altitude, there have been numerous cases of right-ventricle heart failure, with prompt recovery following evacuation to low altitude.

This was described as "human brisket disease" (Anand et al. 1990) in a report about forty afflicted young men about twenty years of age who were all ethnic Garhwalis, Indian soldiers from lowlands south of the Nepalese border. Having been born and raised in the lowlands and coming from a lowland people, these soldiers would be susceptible to the effects of high altitude. Being from a subtropical climate, they would also be severely stressed by their icy posts well above any permanent human habitation, where the nighttime temperatures fall as low as −45°F. Further, their duties required heavy physical exertion, climbing and descending thousands of feet up and down the mountains, carrying supplies, and patrolling the area. Something analogous to brisket disease probably does occur in "susceptible" adult humans if the altitude is high enough and the cold and exercise are extreme.

Today, the continuing research interest relates to human medicine, where progress so often requires that we have an "animal model of a human disease." Insulin was discovered in dogs with diabetes, and cancer treatments are developed using rats with various kinds of tumors. Brisket disease in cattle is a "model" for chronic elevation of pulmonary artery pressure in general, and such elevation complicates nearly all diseases of the heart or lung. But, more specifically, brisket disease is a model for persons, both children and adults, who develop elevated pressures in the lung arteries from exposure to low oxygen.

We now see the full stature of our two scientific pioneers, George Glover and Isaac Newsom. First and foremost, they were intrepid academicians. They had a vision. They lived that vision. It was to expand their modest Colorado Agricultural College into what is now Colorado State University with a fully accredited School of Veterinary Medicine and Biological Sciences. Their contributions to education make them truly outstanding. Yet from the beginning they stressed the importance of scientific research as a vital component of a mature university. It was their research into brisket disease that made them pioneers of altitude research and inspired their "scientific descendants," Rue Jensen, Arch Alexander, and Don Will.

The research of Jensen, Alexander, and Will in turn drew me into the brisket-disease problem and from there into human research at high altitude. The study of the high-school students began decades of research in Leadville, where the St. Vincent's Hospital, run by the Sisters of Charity of Leavenworth, Kansas, became our base. The Sisters were so cooperative that by 1964 we had a fully equipped high-altitude research laboratory in the basement of the hospital. That laboratory became a magnet drawing researchers from all over the country and from around the world. Many aspects of life at high altitude have been studied in Leadville residents, including function of the lung, production of red blood cells, sleep, chronic lung disease, athletic performance, acute altitude sicknesses, pregnancy, and newborn children. Leadville is probably the most completely researched community of high-altitude residents in the world, and the roots of that research can be traced back to Glover and Newsom.

Note

1. R. Jensen, letter to authors, December 20, 1989: "During 1953–1954, Paul Eskridge, Ph.D., physiologist, and I measured pressures in about 15 brisket disease cattle and 10 normal cattle . . . by catheterizing the . . . right heart chambers. At that time I was interested in statistical analysis, but I do not remember analyzing those data. I assume therefore, that the values were obviously higher in affected cattle than in normal cattle and did not require analysis. I have searched without success for the records. So far as I know, those were the first such measurements on brisket cattle."

2

A HIGH POINT IN HUMAN BREATHING

John Scott Haldane of Oxford on Pikes Peak

Piers C. Nye, Ph.D., and John T. Reeves, M.D.

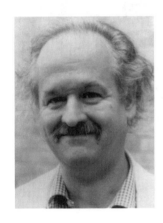

Nye, *left*, and Reeves tell the story of Haldane, the world's foremost pioneer in breathing, and his 1911 expedition to Pikes Peak. Haldane led the Western Hemisphere's first true expedition studying human health at high altitude, and it was a huge success with one glaring exception, which dogged him the rest of his life. Haldane was an outstanding scientist. How, then, did he paint himself into such a corner with his one error? Nye takes the lead in telling the story. He is a lecturer in the University Laboratory of Physiology at Oxford, where Haldane worked. He is also a fellow of Balliol College.

—THE EDITORS

John Scott Haldane (fig. 2.1) was not the first distinguished member of Oxford University to visit Colorado. In 1882, thirty years before him, Oscar Wills O'Flaherty Fingal Wilde, a walking advertisement for Gilbert and Sullivan's light opera *Patience*, had arrived in Leadville "anxious for to shine in the high aesthetic line, as a man of culture rare" (Ellman 1987; Griswold and Griswold 1995). Dressed in a long green overcoat "befrogged and wonderfully befurred" with broad bands of otter skin, with a wide Lord Byron collar and sky blue shirt beneath his large, white, and flat face, he had astounded the Leadville miners both with his wit and with his ability to hold whiskey. The miners were unmoved by his lecture "The Artistic Character of the English Renaissance," but they did honor him by naming a new shaft at Leadville's

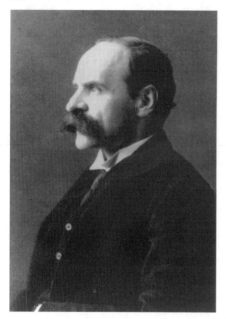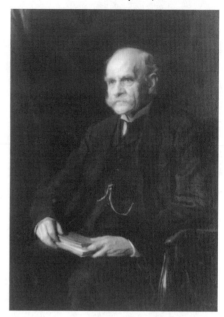

Fig. 2.1. J. S. Haldane. At left is a photograph taken ca 1911. From Cunningham and Lloyd, The Regulation of Human Respiration *(1963), by permission of Blackwell Scientific, Oxford. At right is a portrait of the aged J. S. Haldane by P. A. de Laszlo. (The chain may have supported small gold boxes containing chocolates for his grandchildren.) Courtesy of Scottish National Portrait Gallery.*

Matchless Mine "the Oscar," and they remembered him as "a bully boy with no glass eye."

Wilde's visit had an enormous, if transient, impact—his sayings were telegraphed around the country in advance of his arrival. He advertised *Patience* with great success, his public displays of aestheticism being a necessary preliminary without which the audience would not have understood the subject matter, his own outrageous affectations, that the show satirizes.

Being a scientist and not a famous literary figure, Haldane did not attract such sensationalism, but neither did his visit go unnoticed by the press. On his arrival in July of 1911, the *New York Herald* gave him four column inches, and upon his departure the *New York Times* quadrupled this coverage. Being concerned with a fundamental question of human biology, Haldane left a more lasting and profound mark than did Wilde. In its simplest terms, the question could be written, "How does the body know how much to breathe?" Or put another way, "What controls our breathing?" Though the answer is still not completely known, Haldane seems to have been the first person to ask the question and seriously to seek the answer. In the early years of the twentieth century, seeking the answer led him to Pikes Peak, and that in turn led to his discoveries of altitude acclimatization. In five short weeks on the summit, his varied group (fig. 2.2), Haldane, Douglas[1] from Oxford, Henderson[2] from Yale, and Schneider[3] from Colorado College laid the foundations upon which all subsequent work on acclimatization to high altitude has depended. Haldane's central role in this story, his personality, and the development of his ideas are the subject of this chapter.[4] His single misconception, namely, that the lung membranes actively pump, or secrete, oxygen from the air into the blood, is also considered.

Why would Haldane, in his day the world's greatest expert on breathing, come to Pikes Peak? To answer that question we need to look at the state of knowledge of that day. Scientists understood that, as the body burned fuel to generate heat and energy, oxygen was consumed and a nearly equal volume of carbon dioxide was produced as a byproduct. Breathing thus served two vital functions, supplying oxygen and eliminating carbon dioxide. Before Haldane, till near the end of the nineteenth century, little was known about how human breathing was controlled. When Haldane came on the scene, he began to test the idea that some essential lung function, such as the elimination of carbon dioxide or the uptake of oxygen, might control how much air humans breathed. It was a simple and profound, yet novel, idea.

In the closing years of the nineteenth century, he began his quest by focusing on carbon dioxide. It was known that the body must maintain its normal acid-base balance and that, when dissolved in water or blood, carbon dioxide makes an acid solution. Before the Pikes Peak expedition, Haldane's idea had been that the body automatically adjusts breathing to avoid becoming too acid, or too alkaline. If one breathed "too little," carbon dioxide would be retained within the body and the blood would become acid, which would stimulate an increase in breathing (Zuntz et al. 1860). If one breathed "too much," carbon dioxide would be blown off and the blood would become alkaline, which would inhibit breathing. So perhaps one breathes just enough to maintain acid-base balance. Like many profound ideas it was beautifully simple, and, more than that, it could be tested.

Haldane had developed the methods necessary to estimate non-invasively the level of carbon dioxide in the blood. Being a small and soluble molecule, carbon dioxide moves easily through the tissues. As blood flows through the lung, the molecules pass so quickly from capillary blood into the lung air sacs (the alveoli) that the amount in the blood can be estimated from its concentration in the alveolar air. By taking a sample near the mouth at the end of a full expiration, he obtained air that had come from the alveoli. By using the Haldane apparatus that he had developed, he could measure the carbon dioxide with great accuracy. By simply measuring the carbon dioxide level in the alveolar air, he could monitor the blood level. Today, this procedure is so commonplace that it seems obvious, almost trivial. In Haldane's time it was a major advance, and it also allowed several samples to be taken each minute.

His initial results supported his idea that carbon dioxide controlled breathing. When carbon dioxide levels in resting, normal subjects were measured repeatedly over many months, they were nearly constant, and the values were little different from one subject to the next (Haldane and Priestley 1905). But what about oxygen: did it also have a role to play in controlling breathing? Again, if one breathed too little, as during suffocation, not only would carbon dioxide be retained but concurrently oxygen levels would fall, and this low oxygen, hypoxia, could be an additional stimulus to breathing. So which was the dominant controlling factor, preserving a constant level of carbon dioxide or avoiding hypoxia?

To answer this question, he went to the highest and lowest altitudes at hand in the British Isles. In 1905 he briefly ascended Ben Nevis (4,400 feet; barometric pressure P_B = 646 mm Hg versus sea level = 760 mm Hg) in Scotland, and he descended to the bottom of the Dalcoath Mine in Cornwall (2,240 feet below sea level, P_B ~832 mm Hg). Whereas the oxygen level in air from the lung alveoli fell on ascending Ben Nevis and rose on descending into the mine, the carbon dioxide level hardly changed. These findings supported his view that breathing was apparently regulated to hold the carbon dioxide level constant even though the oxygen level varied. He even entered a compressed-air chamber at London's Brompton Hospital at nearly 2 atmospheres. Again, despite the increase in oxygen, the carbon dioxide level, and therefore the amount of air breathed, remained essentially constant. The results reaffirmed Haldane's belief in the overwhelming power of carbon dioxide (as opposed to oxygen, for example) to control how much air one breathed. But he worried because the exposures were brief and might not tell the whole story.

Three years later, in 1908, when he used longer exposure times in the altitude chamber at the Lister Institute in London, he began to get different results. When he exposed himself for twenty hours to low oxygen in the chamber at a simulated high altitude, there was a substantial fall in his carbon dioxide level, which was still apparent two days after he returned to the normal oxygen environment at sea level (Boycott and Haldane 1908). With a somewhat longer period of reduced oxygen, breathing had increased. Why? Although we now know that, given time, low oxygen stimulates breathing, Haldane leaned toward another explanation. He thought that the low oxygen in the air had caused his body to produce lactic acid, which had caused his breathing to increase. Some decades earlier the great French chemist Pasteur had shown that yeasts deprived of oxygen produced lactic acid. Drawing on Pasteur's finding, Haldane thought that at high altitude lactic acid accumulating within his blood simply increased its acidity, a scheme that fitted well with his conviction that acid drove breathing.

To his credit, Haldane did not let the matter rest there. If his breathing had been stimulated by acid accumulation, he expected breathing to return to normal as the kidney excreted the excess acid over the course of a few days at altitude. In such a case, if he went to high altitude, he expected breathing to increase initially and then over a few days to fall back to the sea-level value even though he remained at altitude. In order to properly test this possible series of events, Haldane wanted exposure to a low-oxygen environment that was longer than could be performed in the Lister Institute's altitude chamber. This is what led him to Pikes Peak.

Haldane wanted an environment suitable for experiments lasting many days and one to which he could transport a large amount of equipment, much of it glassware. His associate, Douglas, had visited Barcroft[5] and the German physiologist Zuntz at the Alta Vista hut at 11,000 feet on Tenerife, one of the Canary Islands, in 1910, but the experiments had not worked well and conditions had severely limited the amount of equipment they could take with them. Some equipment had been modified to make it lighter. These modifications compromised accuracy and contributed to the unsatisfactory results. Haldane's own trip to the summit of Ben Nevis, where he had collected alveolar gas samples, was not remembered fondly. He and his colleagues had been drenched by rain, they had been cold, some glass gas analysis equipment had been broken, and they thought the muscular exercise required to reach the summit had interfered with the results.

At this point in his thinking Haldane met Yandell Henderson of Yale University (fig. 2.2) at the 1910 International Physiological Congress in Vienna. He mentioned to Henderson that he wanted "a nice comfortable, easily accessible, very high mountain with a fairly good hotel on the top," and Henderson replied, "Come to America next summer and we will spend a month or two on Pike's Peak" (Henderson 1938).

The choice of Pikes Peak for the Anglo-American Expedition of 1911 was well considered (Douglas et al. 1913). The altitude of 14,110 feet

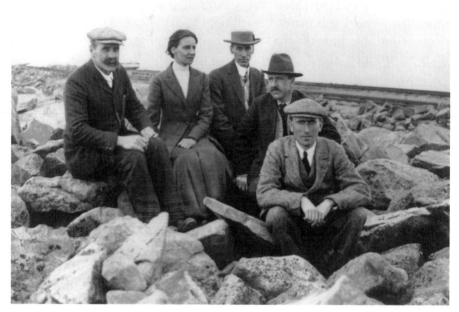

Fig. 2.2. A delayed-action photograph taken by Douglas on the summit of Pikes Peak, 1911. Left to right, J. S. Haldane, Mabel FitzGerald, E. C. Schneider, Y. Henderson, and C. G. Douglas. FitzGerald had interrupted her own studies to come up to the summit for the day. Courtesy the Unviersity Laboratory of Physiology, Oxford.

(barometric pressure P_B = 460 mm Hg) was much higher than Ben Nevis in Scotland, but not so high as to be intolerable. Unlike the Alta Vista hut and Mosso's laboratory on Monte Rosa (14,960 feet) in Italy,[6] Pikes Peak was equipped with a cog railway all the way to the summit. For an expedition, which would require safe transport of some ten large cases of instruments and supplies, such a railway was ideal. On Pikes Peak there would also be a good supply of unacclimatized subjects who would arrive to admire the view but who also would conveniently develop acute mountain sickness. What is more, the employees in the summit house would provide a pool of acclimatized subjects.

Pikes Peak was also within easy reach by rail and telephone of the laboratories at Colorado College in Colorado Springs, fourteen miles away. At the summit was a fifty-yard-long, snow-free track of flat ground that was ideal for exercise studies (fig. 2.3). In addition, the station building had a restaurant and running water. The laboratory where experiments were performed (fig. 2.3) had electricity and was well heated, factors considered important by both Haldane and Douglas. They were all too aware of the extent to which a cold, inhospitable environment and the gloves and bulky clothing that it necessitates can interfere with the accuracy and success of experiments.

It has been said that the primary attraction of Pikes Peak lay in the bodily comforts that it provided. The implication here that Haldane was not a robust man, that he abhorred "roughing it," is manifestly untrue. Douglas (1936) relates that Haldane was renowned for his ability to work productively in mines "under conditions that would have appalled most research workers; it seemed as easy for him to do accurate gas analysis in a cramped attitude by the light of a match or tallow dip as under more comfortable conditions in daylight. [He had] a distressing disregard for lunch, [which] was, after all, but an inconvenience. . . ." Pikes Peak was chosen in preference to the Alps, Andes, Himalayas, and Tenerife for sound practical reasons, not for the easy life that it offered. At the time Pikes Peak was the only place where the process of acclimatization to 14,000 feet could have been properly studied over the course of five weeks.

The findings on Pikes Peak, as well as those by FitzGerald in high-altitude residents (see chap. 3), required that Haldane once again modify his views on the control of breathing. Originally, as noted above, he had thought that breathing would increase only temporarily at high altitude, because of lactic acid accumulation within the body. But the increase in breathing on Pikes Peak was not temporary; rather, to the surprise of Haldane and his colleagues, breathing continued to increase over many days (fig. 2.4). Because the experiments were simple, the methods were tried and true, and because the changes were big and occurred in each subject, there was no doubt of the results. On successive days, as the carbon dioxide level in the air from the lung alveoli progressively fell, the oxygen level rose and the volume of air respired increased. Although lactic acid in the blood was not measured, Haldane felt that lactic acid accumulation could not explain these findings. Having now, for the first time ever, documented the process of acclimatization to altitude, he concluded correctly that the low level of oxygen in the air was somehow stimulating the progressive increase in breathing.

As Haldane revised his ideas about what makes people breathe more at altitude, he developed a comprehensive concept about what determines how much we breathe under a wide variety of conditions. In persons living at sea level, where there is plenty of oxygen available, the body automatically adjusts breathing to defend its acid-base balance by keeping the carbon dioxide level in the blood (and in the lung alveoli) relatively constant. But when one remains for days at high altitude,

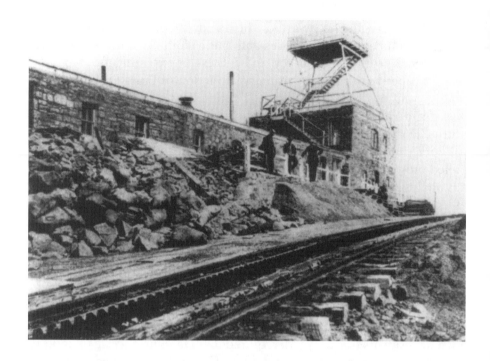

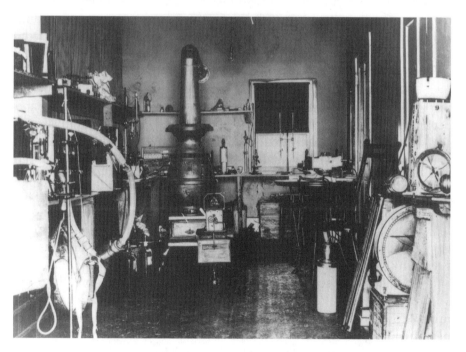

Fig. 2.3. The summit house at Pikes Peak in 1911, showing an exterior view (top) and the laboratory inside (bottom). Haldane's group used the four ground-floor rooms, with private entrance, at the base of the tower. The largest room, lit by electricity and warmed by a wood-burning stove, became their laboratory. Note, at left, a Douglas bag and tubing (for collection of expired air), which largely obscures three sets of Haldane gas analysis equipment. Behind the stove is a galvanometer and, to the right, a circular Fuller's slide rule equivalent to a 25.4-meter straight slide rule. Directly in front of the stove, sitting on a water bath heated from below by a Primus lamp, is a saturator for equilibrating blood with expired gas, required for Haldane's complicated method of measurement of arterial oxygen level. In front of the window are measuring burettes and, to the right, a kymograph for recording events on smoked paper. On top of the box, at right, is the reservoir that supplied controlled drips of water, which displaced pure carbon monoxide from a cylinder. Beside and beneath this box are 1- and 10-liter gasometers to measure gas volumes. The tall white cylinder on the floor contains "oxylith" (sodium peroxide, Na_2O_2), to which water is added for the generation of pure oxygen. Much of this equipment is now in a display assembled by Dan Cunningham, David O'Connor, David Paterson, and Peter Robbins in the University Laboratory of Physiology, Oxford. Reprinted, by permission, from Cunningham, in Respiratory Control *(1989).*

where there is less oxygen in the air, the body acts to defend its oxygen level, and it does this by increasing breathing. But the full increase in breathing cannot occur immediately on arrival at altitude, because the elimination of carbon dioxide (loss of acid) would upset the acid-base balance and cause alkalosis, which would oppose the increase in breathing. Over several days, as the kidney excretes alkali to restore the acid-base balance, breathing progressively increases to a new and higher level. On return to sea level, breathing decreases over several days, for as the carbon dioxide level rises, the kidney must retain alkali to maintain acid-base balance.

What Haldane now understood, and what physiologists still believe, is that levels of *both* oxygen and carbon dioxide are important in controlling how much air we humans breathe. Carbon dioxide is the dominant player over the short term, but over weeks and years oxygen plays the crucial role. Although he had grasped the importance of carbon dioxide in the control of breathing at sea level, he saw clearly the role for oxygen only when he went to Pikes Peak. Not only did Haldane's expedition to Pikes Peak provide us with the first description of the time course of ventilatory acclimatization and "deacclimatization" to high altitude, but also it provided a better understanding of human breathing

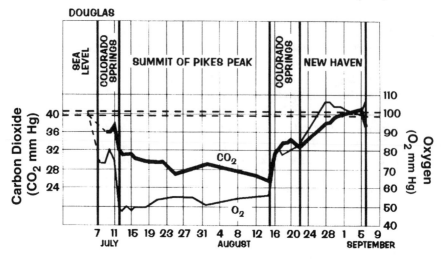

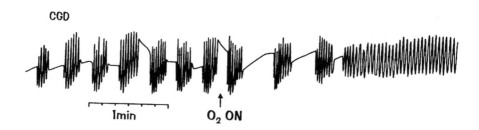

Fig. 2.4. Measurements of breathing in Douglas. The top panel shows levels in alveolar air (measured in mm Hg) of oxygen and carbon dioxide. Arrival on Pikes Peak, July 12, is marked by a sharp fall in oxygen (heavy line) and carbon dioxide (thin line). As ventilation progressively increased, the alveolar levels of carbon dioxide fell further, and oxygen rose. Following descent on August 16 to Colorado Springs and then to New Haven, Connecticut, carbon dioxide and oxygen levels returned to normal sea-level values. The bottom panel shows periodic breathing, which ceases after inspiration of oxygen. The bar indicates one minute. Modified from Douglas et al., Physiological Observations (1913).

in general. Since Haldane's expedition, respiratory and high-altitude physiologists have confirmed his findings on acclimatization, and they continue to struggle to understand how these changes occur. For the mountaineer climbing a high peak, the competitor in an athletic event at altitude, and the skier or tourist in Colorado the basic understanding

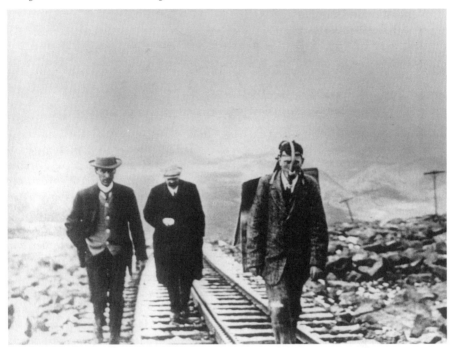

Fig. 2.5. Left to right, *Schneider, Haldane with stopwatch, and Douglas, breathing into bag for measurement of metabolic rate, during exercise on Pikes Peak. Courtesy the University Laboratory of Physiology, Oxford.*

that time is required to increase breathing and blood oxygen levels rests squarely on Haldane's 1911 Pikes Peak expedition.

While people are acclimatizing to altitude, they often suffer distressing irregularities in their breathing pattern, especially during sleep. As Haldane showed, there are repeated episodes of disconcerting deep and rapid breathing followed by many seconds when breathing ceases (fig. 2.4). Although such periodic breathing had been seen occasionally in patients with low oxygen levels at sea level (Pembrey and Allen 1905) and had been noted by Mosso above 14,000 feet on Monte Rosa, Haldane felt that Mosso had not understood the cause. In his attempt to stop periodic breathing, Mosso had administered oxygen through a funnel held close to the face during sleep, but this had not had any effect. Haldane felt that Mosso had used too little oxygen, and so on Pikes Peak he gave a larger flow and found that this quickly brought about return to regular breathing (fig. 2.4). He explained, "Want of oxygen is thus a necessary condition to the production of the periodic breathing." He understood that, in contrast to sea level where carbon dioxide has the overriding role, at altitude the low oxygen now partici-

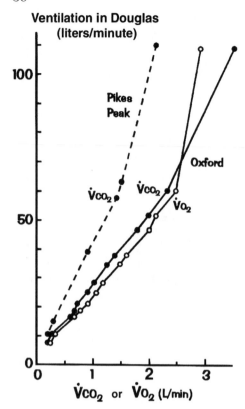

Ventilation in Douglas (liters/minute)

Pikes Peak

Oxford

$\dot{V}CO_2$ $\dot{V}CO_2$ $\dot{V}O_2$

$\dot{V}CO_2$ or $\dot{V}O_2$ (L/min)

Fig. 2.6. *For a given amount of carbon dioxide produced or oxygen consumed during exercise, breathing was much greater on Pikes Peak (dashed line) than in Oxford (unbroken lines). As the exercise became severe, the lines became steeper, and Haldane correctly speculated that muscle release of lactic acid provided an additional stimulus to breathing. He also suggested that lactic acid would be more easily released in a low-oxygen environment than at sea level. Modified from Cunningham and Lloyd,* The Regulation of Respiration *(1963).*

pates more actively in the moment-to-moment control of breathing. At high altitude when both oxygen and carbon dioxide levels are low but the body has not fully acclimatized, these two regulators have opposing influences on breathing and can easily get out of step with each other, causing, as he said, "this violent game of battledore-and-shuttlecock[7] . . . in the respiratory centre."

When we go to high altitude, our most prominent sensation is breathlessness during exercise, and Haldane on Pikes Peak was the first to examine this in detail (fig. 2.5). Near sea level in Oxford, his laboratory had already shown for the first time (1905) that increases in work performed during moderate exercise were matched perfectly by increases in the body's requirement for oxygen, the amount of carbon dioxide expelled, and the amount of air breathed (fig. 2.6). These all seemed to be in lockstep with each other. But when the exercise became severe, the lockstep was broken, for breathing began to increase more sharply. If severe exertion caused the exercising muscles to release an acid (such as lactic acid) into the blood, this would account for the additional stimulus to breathing. Although Haldane didn't measure lactic acid, he did speculate that it would increase. "During sudden and severe muscular exertion the circulation through the active muscles is insufficient to supply them with all the oxygen they require . . . [and] some lactic acid is formed." Once again he was correct, as confirmed years later by Dill's group at Harvard (see chap. 5).

On Pikes Peak, even with mild exercise, he found that breathing was strikingly enhanced and was almost twice that at sea level (fig. 2.6). As to why exercise should increase breathing so much at high altitude, he speculated that exercise had caused the oxygen level in the arterial blood to fall below the one at rest and furthermore that the exercising muscles produced more lactic acid at altitude than at sea level. Even though he could not measure the levels of either arterial oxygen or lactic acid during exercise, both speculations were proved to be correct by subsequent investigators (chap. 5).

Well before Pikes Peak, scientists knew that the number of red cells and the hemoglobin concentration in a sample of blood increase at high altitude, a response that helps the blood carry more oxygen. Although the reason usually given had been that the reduced amount of oxygen at high altitude caused the bone marrow to make more red cells, there was an additional possibility. If water left the blood at altitude, then the blood would be more concentrated, and the red blood cell count and the hemoglobin concentration would increase even if no new cells entered the circulation. We now know that many days are required to produce enough new red blood cells to cause a large increase in their total number within the body. Haldane must have suspected this, because he made repeated measurements of the total amount of hemoglobin (calculated from blood volume) in the body, and he could do this by breathing a known amount of carbon monoxide (see appendix). During the first week on the summit, the blood hemoglobin concentration rose as expected, but the blood volume fell. Now for the first time the initial rise in hemoglobin concentration at altitude could be attributed to a rapid loss of water from the blood (Douglas et al. 1913). Over the ensuing weeks blood volume returned toward normal as new red blood cells entered the circulation. While the production of new red cells is a slow process, the body cleverly increases hemoglobin concentration soon after arrival at altitude by removing water from the blood, a concept that goes back to Haldane.

Blood oxygen level, concentration of hemoglobin, and blood volume—all affect how much blood the heart pumps each minute, a measurement known as cardiac output. But in 1911 an accurate measurement of cardiac output in humans was not possible. So Haldane and company estimated output by indirect methods and were surprised by how little change they found in acclimatized subjects. These results were later confirmed in 1929 on Pikes Peak by Grollman (see chap. 4), who used his more reliable acetylene method for measuring cardiac output. Haldane marveled that acclimatization to high altitude should result in such a large increase in ventilation with so little change in circulation.

For some time, Haldane and Douglas had been wondering about the relative roles of lowered carbon dioxide versus lowered oxygen in causing altitude sickness that was known to occur often soon after ascent. On Tenerife in 1910 the observations by Douglas and Barcroft had suggested that low oxygen was more likely to cause symptoms than was low carbon dioxide. For example, Barcroft, who suffered greatly from altitude sickness, increased his breathing only slightly, which resulted in severe hypoxia but little change in his carbon dioxide. By contrast, Douglas, who remained well, had a large increase in breathing, which helped maintain his oxygen level but lowered his carbon dioxide. Thus low oxygen, but not low carbon dioxide, seemed to be the key factor. On Pikes Peak, similar results were obtained. Henderson, who suffered least from mountain sickness, breathed most vigorously, whereas Schneider, who suffered "intense frontal headache, nausea and sleeplessness for the better part of a week," breathed least. Surprisingly, the alkalosis from the low carbon dioxide appeared to make little, if any, contribution to the development of mountain sickness. This conclusion was also supported by Grollman (see chap. 4), but it is only now becoming widely accepted.

The findings on Pikes Peak led Haldane to suggest the use of oxygen for the treatment of mountain sickness, especially "pneumonia . . . , [which] is very dangerous at high altitude." The pneumonia referred to was presumably high-altitude pulmonary edema (see chap. 7). Haldane suggested that oxygen levels might also be raised by the use of pressurized chambers or by breathing small amounts of carbon dioxide to stimulate ventilation, and both methods have subsequently been shown to be effective. Haldane (1917a) also pioneered oxygen therapy for the treatment of victims of gas warfare in World War I.

Taken together, these were remarkable new findings and new concepts. Haldane and company found that residing on Pikes Peak caused breathing to be set at a new and higher level. The process required several days, during which time carbon dioxide levels progressively fell and oxygen levels progressively rose. Before the process was complete, breathing was often disorganized and intermittent, no matter whether the subjects were resting, had finished exercise, or were asleep. Oxygen lack contributed to this disorganized breathing, and not lack of

carbon dioxide only, as had been previously supposed. Following acclimatization, exercise of a given intensity required just as much oxygen
as at sea level, but the breathing required was much greater. They found
that on Pikes Peak blood hemoglobin rose in two steps. The first was
simply a concentrating of the red cells as water was lost from the blood.
The second step was much slower; total hemoglobin in the body increased as new red blood cells entered the circulation. They correctly
guessed from imprecise measurements that the amount of blood pumped
by the heart increased only temporarily on arrival on the Peak. They
also concluded that acute altitude sicknesses resulted from oxygen lack
and not from reduced carbon dioxide as some had previously thought.
Finally, they correctly predicted that a fully acclimatized person might
just be able to reach the summit of Mt. Everest (29,028 feet) without
supplementary oxygen. It was a large number of remarkable new findings, and the conclusions have stood the test of time. No wonder their
published report was 134 pages long.

Had Haldane been content with the findings so far, his expedition
would have been hailed universally as an unqualified success, and he
would have been spared considerable criticism. But it was not to be. He
had a second reason, which was, subconsciously perhaps, the driving
force for going to Pikes Peak. He wanted to prove a theory that was
haunting him, namely, that when the body was in need of oxygen, the
lung membranes actively pumped, or, as he said, "secreted," oxygen
from the alveolar air into the blood. He realized full well that here he
was swimming upstream against the current of medical opinion. In a
nonliving system, when there are many oxygen molecules on one side
of a porous membrane and fewer on the other, oxygen molecules move
across the membrane so that in time the numbers on each side equalize.
Oxygen molecules, in effect, flow downhill from a higher to a lower
partial pressure in a passive process called diffusion. Most physiologists believed then (and still do) that oxygen moves passively by diffusion from the alveolar air spaces across the lung's membranes into the
blood, just as carbon dioxide moves passively in the other direction. But
Haldane felt strongly that a reduction in the amount of oxygen available to human beings could cause lung membranes to actively secrete
(actively pump) oxygen from the air into the blood. This, then, was his
search—to find a condition that unequivocally would bring out the active secretion of oxygen from lungs to blood. He thought the proper
conditions for oxygen secretion might exist at high altitude, and a good
test of the idea could be conducted on Pikes Peak.

His problem was to measure oxygen on both sides of the lung membranes—in the alveolar air and in the blood. The alveolar side was not

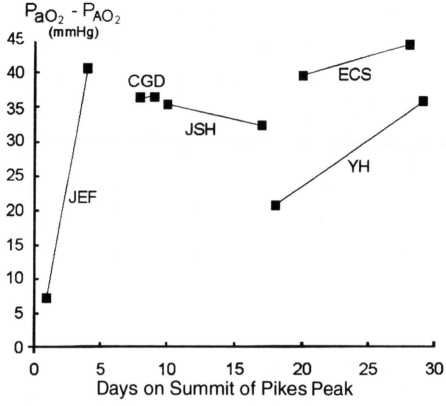

Fig. 2.7. *Using his carbon monoxide method, Haldane found that the oxygen level (measured as oxygen pressure) was higher in the arterial blood (PaO_2) than in the alveolar air (PAO_2), leading to his claim that lung membranes actively "secreted" (pumped) oxygen from air to blood. Haldane found "secretion" was relatively small when J. E. Fuller, a Colorado Springs resident, arrived on Pikes Peak, but was large after several days' residence at altitude in Fuller and in the four scientists themselves. Drawn from data in Douglas 1913.*

an issue; he had mastered that. The problem was to measure it on the other side—in the blood, and arterial blood would do. If oxygen pressure in the alveoli of the lung was always higher than that in the arterial blood, then oxygen could be transferred across the lung membrane passively, that is, by diffusion alone. But if the pressure of arterial oxygen, under any circumstance, was higher than alveolar oxygen, something more elaborate than simple diffusion must be helping it along—oxygen must be actively secreted (pumped) from alveolar air to blood.

Because at the time it was not thought possible to take samples of blood directly from human arteries, he developed an ingenious, yet indirect and complicated, way of measuring oxygen in arterial blood (Haldane 1896, Douglas 1912). The method made use of his discoveries that oxygen and carbon monoxide competed with each other very precisely in combining with hemoglobin. The competition is like the children's game King of the Mountain; increasing oxygen will shove carbon monoxide off hemoglobin, but increasing carbon monoxide will displace the oxygen. Haldane's early experiments using his carbon monoxide method gave alarmingly high values for the pressure of oxygen in the arterial blood, values three or even four times those of alveolar air (Smith and Haldane 1897). These extraordinary results led him to believe that oxygen must be secreted from the alveoli into pulmonary capillary blood. The belief was reinforced by the knowledge that many fish and single-celled organisms actively secrete (pump) oxygen into their swim bladders against a very high oxygen pressure gradient.

He soon discovered that his method incorporated many pitfalls. If the temperature or carbon dioxide level were low, if he did the experiments in artificial light rather than daylight, if there was contamination by bacteria, or if he didn't allow enough time for carbon monoxide to diffuse into blood, the results were in error. Most of the errors gave oxygen levels in arterial blood that were too high. But instead of looking for a completely different technique, he made successive refinements to his own method until he was confident he had eliminated the potential errors in the method and that it was accurate. The method and his confidence in it were to bring him to grief.

Using his complicated method, Haldane and his colleagues obtained results that not only, they felt, supported their hypothesis, but also exceeded their expectations. At sea level in Oxford, when they briefly breathed a low-oxygen mixture, they had found oxygen levels in blood close to those in the alveolar air, that is, little evidence of secretion. But after several days on Pikes Peak, their results indicated much higher oxygen levels in the blood than in the lung air, indicating to them that oxygen had been pumped (secreted) from the air into the blood. Furthermore, the finding was consistent in all nine experiments in five subjects (fig. 2.7). Haldane felt he had proven his hypothesis. Not only that, but the effect was so large that the oxygen level in the arterial blood had returned essentially to that found at sea level!

In his experimental findings on Pikes Peak there was an unusually cruel stroke of fate. In the one subject studied within an hour of arrival at the summit of Pikes Peak, Haldane found a low oxygen level in the arterial blood, in effect, little or no "oxygen secretion." Yet, after four days' residence on the Peak, this subject's level had risen to match those of Haldane's party who were residing there (fig. 2.7), suggesting that his lungs had developed the ability to secrete oxygen into the blood over four days at high altitude. As a result, Haldane came to believe that the acclimatization process not only involved an increase in breathing, but also that lung membranes progressively developed the capacity to pump oxygen into the blood. This stroke of fate sealed Haldane's conviction that the lungs developed the power to secrete oxygen into the blood when most needed, but here his faith in the supreme accuracy of his techniques had let him down.

Given that Haldane proposed an "oxygen secretion" so powerful that it raised the oxygen level on Pikes Peak to that at sea level, the question has been repeatedly asked how he could believe his amazing results. He did have the occasional qualm about the idea that these very thin membranes of the lung could secrete so much oxygen. Furthermore, if blood oxygen levels on Pikes Peak were as high as at sea level, it was odd that the hemoglobin and ventilation would rise so much. And he should have been more concerned over the vast amount of energy required to pump all this oxygen "uphill," from a lower to a higher pressure. He reassured himself with the fact that, although the faces and lips of new arrivals at the summit were blue, both became red during acclimatization as the saturation of hemoglobin rose. The blueness of new arrivals he reported was used forcefully by the Kroghs[8] (Schmidt-Nielson 1995) as evidence for the lack of secretion, but they overlooked Haldane's claim that secretion increases only gradually as acclimatization occurs. Nevertheless, Haldane should have listened to these doubts that arose within himself and in the minds of other scientists.

It wasn't many years before the scientific community had refuted Haldane's oxygen secretion theory. When it became possible to insert a needle into a human artery, arterial blood oxygen levels were measured directly and were found to be slightly lower than those in the alveolar air and not higher, as Haldane had proposed. Clearly, there was no oxygen secretion by the lung membranes. Such were the conclusions of Barcroft's 1921 expedition to Cerro de Pasco, Peru, and Dill's 1929 expedition to Leadville (chap. 5).

What had Haldane done wrong? Although in this one instance he was wrong, it is not clear why he was wrong. Not only did Haldane stake his reputation on these findings from Pikes Peak, but also, as we shall see, he stubbornly clung to his "oxygen secretion" theory until he died. Perhaps he had based his conclusions upon what might today be considered a dangerously small sample size. But if he had used a statistical test, it would have given him a probability of a million to one, supporting his conclusions. The explanation must involve an error in method that became augmented at altitude and possibly during the course of acclimatization. But whatever the explanation, Haldane's error remains a mystery to this day.

Who was this brilliant and complicated man? Understanding why a prominent Oxford scientist would want to leave the cultured environment of Victorian England for the rarified air of Pikes Peak nearly one hundred years ago and why he would be willing to risk his reputation on a controversial theory requires, first of all, an understanding of his brilliant and rather eccentric family. Perhaps if one comes from, and gives rise to, individuals of truly extraordinary accomplishment, this creates expectations not only from others but, more importantly, from within oneself.

Born into the Scottish aristocracy in May 1860, Haldane had ancestors and descendants who were leaders in military, political, and academic affairs of the country. The Haldanes had been robust men of war based at Gleneagles, which is now famous for its hotel and golf course but was then in the path of tribal highlanders who came down to raid cattle in the richer lowlands. In the seventeenth century John Haldane, a great-great-great-great-grandfather, was a Scottish representative with Cromwell's army during the civil war.

The family was not only robust, but it also contained a doggedly righteous streak. For example, J.S.H.'s maternal grandfather (Burdon Sanderson) persuaded his daughter Mary, on religious grounds, to break off her first marriage "for the sake of her soul" and to marry a "dry Scotch widower with five children." This was Robert Haldane, who proposed to Mary over his wife's grave and with whom he had five more children. J. S., the second of these, therefore had nine siblings and half siblings. One sibling, Elizabeth, wrote several books, including a *Life of Descartes*, and she became Scotland's first woman justice of the peace.

Haldane's elder brother, Richard (1856–1928), the Right Honorable Viscount Haldane of Cloan, Fellow of the Royal Society O.M., "so incredibly urbane as to be almost a character in a French play," became, appropriately, secretary of state for war under Asquith and later lord chancellor under the first Labour government. He started the Territorial Army and the Continental Expeditionary Force, which together are said to have prevented Britain from succumbing to the Germans in the early stages of World War I. He also set up the Officer Training Corps for schoolboys and university students and translated writings of the German philosopher Schopenhauer.

Intellectual pursuits, including experimental medicine, ran strongly in the family. John Burdon Sanderson, Haldane's uncle and professor of physiology at Oxford, had fought off the antivivisectionist lobby and had established the University Laboratory of Physiology in 1884, one year after Haldane had graduated in medicine at Edinburgh University. J. S. Haldane's son, J.B.S. Haldane, a brilliant writer of popular biological and political essays, was better known to the general public. His fame was enhanced and sustained by the pleasure he took in shocking those around him. A notorious, but not untypical, example of his alarming eccentricity was his insistence that those under him in an experimental "bomb factory" in the World War I trenches should all smoke cigarettes while they worked. At the same time the mere possession of a clay pipe or tobacco by a worker at Waltham Abbey, Britain's largest explosives factory, resulted in immediate dismissal. He explained his rule "on psychological grounds, as I thought it important that we should have absolute confidence in one another and in our weapons" (Clark 1968). J.B.S.'s real fame stems from his reconciliation of Mendelian genetics with Darwinian theory, thereby founding neo-Darwinism and population genetics. Peter Medawar (1968) described him as the "grand master of modern evolution theory."

J. S. Haldane's daughter, the late Naomi Mitchison, C.B.E. (commander of the British Empire), best known as a historical novelist, wrote over eighty books on subjects ranging from Socrates to Alfred the Great, from birth control to oil in the Scottish Highlands, from African history to children's stories, from science fiction to romantic poetry. She also wrote two acclaimed autobiographies. She sat on the Highlands and Islands Advisory Panel. She was tribal mother to the Bakgatla tribe in Botswana and was the dedicatee of J. D. Watson's *The Double Helix* (1968). Naomi's three sons, all professors of biological sciences, are listed in *Who's Who*. One of Naomi's daughters, Lois, published in 1966 during the Cultural Revolution a book on China and has been far eastern correspondent for the *Manchester Guardian* newspaper. Her other daughter, Rosalind, has written twelve books on various subjects, such as *Eighteenth-Century Scottish History*, *Sexuality and Social Control*, and *Coping with Destitution: Poverty and Relief in Western Europe*.

Naomi died in 1999, aged 101, and was surely the oldest person to have a personal home page on the Internet (contributed by American feminist admirers). She remembered the day in 1911 when Haldane and Douglas set out for Pikes Peak. The family, in typically challenging, if mistaken, Haldane style, expressed skepticism at the idea of rejecting Scottish mountains in favor of American ones. "They are no larger in Colorado," one disparaging family member remarked, "it's just that they start higher up!"

Haldane and his wife, Kathleen, lived largely separate lives. He had his own end of the house for writing and experiments. Kathleen had little appreciation of his eminence, partly because she did not understand his science and partly because, unlike his elder brother, Viscount Haldane, and members of her own, much-knighted family, he was not a distinguished political figure. She was a high-imperialist Tory, whereas he was liberal, with very different views on subjects such as the Boer War. Home life was enlivened by the presence of a Scottish terrier and an assertive, free-range macaw inherited, at the age of forty, from Kathleen's family, who could no longer tolerate its screams. There were numerous other animals, including ducks and the occasional cat that, according to Kathleen's autobiography (1961), followed Haldane home from the laboratory.

Haldane put a lot of time into the upbringing and education of his children and grandchildren, and he was very popular with them. Not only did his own life show the excitement of academic pursuits, but he demonstrated to them how, on occasion, the excitement can be enhanced by danger. For example, he introduced his son, Jack (J.B.S. Haldane), at the age of seven to the "gentle and surreptitious power of hypoxia" by asking him to climb to a hypoxic region in a mine to recite "Friends, Romans, Countrymen, lend me . . ." He failed to reach "your ears." Jack was also submerged in leaky diving suits, far too big for him, at a very young age.

In later years Naomi's children stayed with him frequently. This was partly because his house (now demolished to make way for Oxford University's Wolfson College) was next to the school they attended. On each end of a watch chain hanging from his waistcoat was a small golden box that always contained a chocolate for them. Having received such an extraordinarily generous helping of both genes and environment, his children and grandchildren, not surprisingly, have led distinguished lives.

With such an accomplished family, Haldane could be expected to have a many-faceted, and even complex, personality. Although he was a courteous and rather formal man, who was known by all who worked with him as the "Senior Partner," he had no time for the formality of London's gentlemen's clubs. Shortly after Haldane's marriage, his uncle, Professor Burdon Sanderson, put his name down for one of the most distinguished of these, the Athenaeum. But Haldane soon resigned, explaining that he had no use for a place where his mining colleagues would not be welcome as guests for lunch. New College at Oxford appears to have been more welcoming. His working habits were demanding of himself and of his associates. Having worked through much of the night, he would arrive at the laboratory, fresh from his breakfast, at about midday. This lifestyle did not fit in well with that of his subordinates, "whose humbler tasks necessitated getting up at a more orthodox hour" (Douglas 1936). On Pikes Peak, when he realized that their 6:00 A.M. start of the working day coincided with Oxford's afternoon, things improved for all.

A many-faceted, complicated personality was reflected in his philosophy both of life and of science. In his earliest publications, "The Relation of Philosophy to Science" and "Life and Mechanism" (in *Nature,* 1960), produced at the age of twenty-three and twenty-four, he indicated that biology was far more complex than the sciences of physics and chemistry. Feeling that biology dealt with a coordinated whole not entirely explained by the known laws of physics and chemistry, he favored a more holistic approach than that of the mechanists (Mayr 1997). He felt it wrongheaded to liken a body to a machine, which is separate from the environment and is continually worn down by use. In response to its environment, an organism can remake or repair itself as when damaged blood vessels become normal again, tissue swelling disappears, or cut nerves regenerate. And of course there was the gradual and exquisitely tuned acclimatization to high altitude (Haldane 1917b). In rejecting mechanistic explanations, he commented that here "it is life, not matter which we have before us."

Such a statement may appear to suggest that Haldane felt that a "vital principle" differentiated life from matter. Indeed, as already indicated, he felt that breathing regulated the acid-base balance of the body with a "marvelous exactitude" as though there was guidance "by an outside agency, just as a locomotive is guided by the driver." Yet he rejected vitalism when he argued that his own experiments showed that carbon dioxide provided the necessary signal for breathing. No supernatural driver was needed here, only equipment sensitive enough to detect small changes in carbon dioxide. Even a mind as brilliant as Haldane's could not foresee the enormous advances of biochemistry, molecular biology, and genetics, yet he understood well that layers of complexity not seen in the nonliving world are needed to explain living processes.

Further insight into Haldane's personality comes from his anonymous eight-thousand-word *Letter to Edinburgh Professors* (1890). As a medical student, Haldane had not enjoyed the course at Edinburgh. It had emphasized "facts, rules-of-thumb, practical tips and other odds and ends while ignoring the experimental observations and reasonings on which they are based." His failure in one medical examination triggered, some years later, the letter, which lambasted the fact-based course for "plunging [students] into a region of intellectual darkness, in which we were left without a clue," and for its use of a third-rate textbook, "whose muddle-headedness would astound any one whose sense of wonder had not been already blunted by looking into the minds of text book writers and lecturers." He complained of examinations that promoted success among the mindless, but "well trained, professional prize-takers." He attacked "illusory, so called practical classes which were of no more 'practical' advantage to the students . . . than if they were made to turn a handle for an hour daily."

The letter ends with a call to the professors: "Let them rouse themselves! Let them plainly denounce the humbug which has for a time got the upper hand around them! They will have the enthusiastic support of those who feel the blighting influence of the present system of teaching, who feel that that system is utterly unworthy of a school with such a tradition as ours." While this splendid letter would ring true for, and give heart to, many of today's oppressed medical students, it was not all diatribe, for it contained constructive suggestions on how the course could be improved. In 1890 the letter was published and sold for sixpence.

For Haldane, the letter was not a sterile academic exercise, but an expression of principles that guided his life. Upon graduating from Edinburgh, he immediately put his ideas to the test about the need to make "reasonings based on experimental observations." He accepted a job as a demonstrator (roughly equivalent to an assistant professor in the United States) in Dundee, Scotland, where he studied the bacterial and chemical composition of air in local houses, schools, and sewers. From these early observations of those working in confined spaces where the immediate environment can threaten well-being or safety, he set the tone for a career that remained centered firmly on a desire to understand and improve working conditions (Passmore 1963). He was particularly concerned about miners, divers, submariners, and factory workers. The latter breathed the hot, foul air of factories owned by the captains of industry who, all too often, put profit before humanity in their desperate attempt to join the upper classes. Although Haldane was not overtly left-wing, his goals were entirely complementary to those of the left. And although he came from a long line of Scottish aristocrats, he was an ardent liberal who wanted to increase the workingman's quality of life as well as increase productivity. As we shall see, in both of these goals he was spectacularly successful.

If a long train of remarkable scientific successes (see appendix) confirms one's confidence in the ability to do good science, then perhaps we can begin to understand why Haldane argued so strongly in defense of his "oxygen secretion" theory. From his beginning as a scientist everything seemed to go right. At the outset the crucial measurement in confined, polluted environments was the chemical composition of the air that the workers breathed. One of Haldane's strengths was to develop new and accurate techniques to measure the composition of air. These soon became standard throughout the world, and several remained so for fifty years. The Haldane (now Lloyd-Haldane) gas analyzer reliably measured the carbon dioxide and oxygen in the air in various environments to the remarkable accuracy of about one part in seven thousand.

Using this analyzer he showed that the foulness of air (chokedamp), which caused the occasional fatality among those who repaired wells in England, resulted from a deficiency of oxygen and not, as had been previously supposed, from an excess of carbon dioxide or from the presence of poisonous gases (1896a). When barometric pressure was low or falling, foul air issued from the surrounding strata where oxidation of iron had removed oxygen. Thus, wells were usually safe when the weather was fine, but they could be dangerous when it was unsettled. Because the danger in wells arose simply from oxygen lack, diminution in the flame of a household candle could be a useful warning of danger. Normally, air contains 21 percent oxygen, and a candle flame becomes notably smaller at 17 percent, a level that is well tolerated by humans. But a candle flame is not useful in mines where poisonous and explosive gases are likely to be found (1896b). Early on his careful measurements made for good science, which in turn improved the workplace.

In the long run Haldane's successes with carbon monoxide also enormously benefited the workingman. He reported to the secretary of state for the Home Department (1896b) on the causes of death of fifty-seven miners and thirty horses in an explosion in the Tylorstown colliery. Previously, the common view was that death, from causes other than explosion, resulted from breathing blackdamp, which is air deficient in oxygen and containing an excess of carbon dioxide. Haldane's analysis of blood from the dead men showed that fifty-two of the fifty-seven men had some 80 percent of their hemoglobin bound by carbon monoxide, meaning that they must have been breathing for a long time after the explosion and that death had resulted from carbon monoxide poisoning, not deficiency of oxygen or excess of carbon dioxide. To prove his point, he showed that carbon monoxide binds much more avidly to hemoglobin than does oxygen, and breathing air containing only 0.1 percent carbon monoxide eventually excludes oxygen and is fatal. Because carbon monoxide poisoning causes oxygen deficiency, the symptoms of euphoria and lethargy as poisoning develops are indistinguishable from those of oxygen lack experienced by balloonists and mountaineers at extreme altitudes, a subject he was familiar with from Paul Bert's book *La Pression barométrique*.[9]

His work showed that the preference of hemoglobin for carbon monoxide was more than 150 times that for oxygen. Even worse, when large amounts of carbon monoxide were present in the blood, hemoglobin could scarcely release to the cells even the oxygen that it contained, indicating that carbon monoxide poisoning was more vicious than severe anemia. In these studies Haldane didn't spare himself. In one experiment, he reached a carbon monoxide saturation of 56 percent, at which point he stopped the experiment because of "palpitations, giddiness and dullness of the senses. . . . I could hardly stand, and could not walk alone without falling down" (Haldane 1895). It was in this condition that he was once detained by the police on his way home from the laboratory. On another occasion he was seen by his housekeeper, who consoled Kathleen by saying, "I know's how you feel ma'am, my husband's just the same on a Friday night."

Based on his understanding that small animals with their high metabolism succumb to carbon monoxide and other forms of oxygen lack in about one-twentieth the time required for humans, Haldane introduced caged mice and canaries to mines and submarines, where their behavior gave many minutes' warning of impending danger. Whereas miners and submariners had previously relied on candles or the flames of their lamps to indicate the presence of hypoxic areas, he showed that these were useless for the detection of lethal amounts of carbon monoxide. Another practical application he suggested was the use of carbon monoxide gas for the destruction of plague-infected rats on ships. His work led from one advance to another, and many of them brought practical benefit to the working individual.

Long before Haldane went to Pikes Peak, where the barometric pressure was low, he had become interested in the effects on humans of *high* barometric pressures (Donald 1963). He was concerned about the well-being of divers and of men working in pressurized diving bells, called caissons, while building the foundations of bridges or tunnels through water-bearing strata. Because suits were often poorly ventilated with fresh air during a dive, Haldane knew that the men would be faced with a buildup of carbon dioxide. Although the buildup would be well tolerated for very shallow dives, the divers would be at risk of narcosis caused by high carbon dioxide levels while working at great depths. If dangerous narcosis were to be avoided, the ventilation of a diver's suit must be increased as he goes deeper, or a carbon dioxide absorber must be included in the breathing circuit.

In Haldane's day, divers and caisson workers suffered much from the "bends," a painful condition on resurfacing that caused disability or even death. Because nearly 80 percent of the atmosphere is nitrogen, large quantities of it would be driven into the tissues of men working under high pressures, and he reasoned correctly that, as a diver ascends from depth, nitrogen bubbles forming in tissues and released into the bloodstream would cause bends. Oxygen could not be implicated because it is rapidly consumed by the tissues, nor could carbon dioxide, because it is so soluble. Having performed experiments on goats that determined how nitrogen under high pressure was driven into the tissues, he was able to draw up the first effective tables of decompression times for the prevention of bends. Ascent was in stages, starting with large reductions in absolute pressure and, as the diver approached the surface, with small reductions. Although his tables were published in 1908 (Boycott et al. 1908), more than ninety years ago, they have been little improved upon since.

Because nitrogen is poorly soluble, it is only slowly taken up by the tissues during a dive, which means one can safely ascend back to the surface rather quickly after brief dives lasting, say, for less than twenty minutes. Divers making a slow descent—thought at the time to reduce the likelihood of the bends—only made things worse because it gave their tissues more time to load up with nitrogen. If the Eustachian tubes to the ears remained open, Haldane found that speeding up the rate of descent twenty- or even fortyfold could be achieved safely. With these two changes in the customary practice, that is, rapid descent and ascent by stages, the amount of time available for work on the bottom was greatly increased. Not only had Haldane shown how health and safety concerns increased, rather than impaired, productivity, but also he showed that his concern for the welfare of workingmen led to better scientific knowledge.

Haldane also experimented in collaboration with his son, J.B.S. Haldane, with early forms of the self-contained Aqua-lung, for which the French underwater explorer Jacques Cousteau later perfected a valve. With Haldane's model, many hundreds of divers recovered in World War I enemy mines from harbors at depths down to 150 feet. He stated that none of these "frogmen" lost his life for a "physiological reason," meaning presumably that no lives were lost because of straightforward failure of his apparatus.

Remarkably, in 1933 Haldane built and tested the first space suit. He did so in response to a request from Mark Ridge, an American who wanted to use one for ballooning to extreme altitudes. Ridge had been refused, for safety reasons, permission to try out a "spacesuit" in the United States, but Haldane persuaded Sir Robert Davis, maker of England's finest diving suits, to make appropriate modifications to one of his products. In this pressurized suit and without complication, they took Ridge, breathing 100 percent oxygen to avoid the bends, down to the lowest achievable chamber pressure, 17 mm Hg, equivalent to an altitude of about 100,000 feet. Haldane concluded, "These experiments show quite clearly that the dress could be used for either balloon or aeroplane ascents without any limit to the height attainable with safety."

Haldane continued his scientific explorations near to the end of his life. Having shown that a large mass of broken coal could ignite spontaneously, he investigated in his later years the causes of fires in haystacks (Haldane and Makgill 1923). Much to the amusement of his grandchildren, he plunged thermometers deep into damp stacks to discover whether or not spontaneously generated heat could ignite the hay. In a sufficiently large haystack, he concluded, the buildup of heat from chemical oxidation could run out of control and result in spontaneous combustion. Elephants and whales have avoided this problem by evolving a low metabolism, an option not available to haystacks (Smith 1985).

In his seventies (fig. 2.1) he published work on atmospheric pollution and fogs, silicosis in coal miners, the passage of water and gases through human skin, the therapeutic use of oxygen and carbon dioxide, the treatment of burns after colliery explosions, the energetics of mining coal, color vision, philosophy, and science and religion. At the age of seventy-five, one year before his death, he also produced, with J. G. Priestley, the second edition of his great textbook *Respiration* (1935). He then traveled to Iran to investigate heatstroke in oil refineries. He died at midnight on March 14–15, 1936, shortly after his return from Iran.

To the end Haldane retained his belief in oxygen secretion by the lungs at high altitude, as indicated by a quote from the 1935 edition of *Respiration*. "One of the objects of this [Pikes Peak] expedition was to determine whether the want of oxygen . . . at 14,000 feet [produced] active secretion of oxygen inwards. The method . . . was employed with every precaution against errors. The results obtained were quite unmistakable . . . as soon as acclimatization . . . was established the 'arterial' oxygen pressure became considerably higher than that of the alveolar air."

Why did Haldane hold on so tenaciously to the idea of oxygen secretion? Perhaps it was the family's doggedly righteous streak. But such an explanation is not entirely satisfactory. Doggedly righteous he may have been, but his own results could convince him to change his opinion. For example, on Pikes Peak he revised his ideas on breathing to include a controlling role for oxygen, whereas before this he had been convinced that the acidity from carbon dioxide was *the* regulator. If he had continued to work on oxygen secretion, he might well have come to the correct conclusion there too. Perhaps the appropriate question is, "Why did he stop working on the secretion issue?" Of course the Great War of 1914–1918 intervened, but even afterward he did not return to experiments on secretion. Sorting out the problem would have been a dispiriting task, and the necessary experiments might have required a laboratory and equipment not readily available to him.

Scientific opinion was weighted against Haldane. In 1910 August and Marie Krogh of Copenhagen had published in English a series of papers that severely criticized the idea of the lung actively "secreting" oxygen into the blood. This criticism had been reinforced when August Krogh came, at Haldane's invitation, to a meeting of the British Medical Association in 1910. There Krogh demonstrated his methods and described results that he and his wife, Marie, had obtained opposing Haldane's theory. Then in 1915, Marie Krogh used Haldane's own carbon monoxide rebreathing procedure to show that the diffusion of oxygen across the lung membranes was large enough that there was no need to invoke oxygen secretion. These events, though not affecting the friendship that Haldane and Krogh held with each other, were very damaging to Haldane's theory.

Haldane's cherished goal was to become the Waynflete professor of physiology at Oxford and head of the laboratory that his own uncle had established. In 1913 he was one of two candidates for the chair, but there was an element of bad timing in this. No candidate for the job ever came up against more distinguished competition. The neurophysiologist Sherrington,[10] the other candidate, was already regarded as a great man. Also, there was widespread skepticism of Haldane's oxygen secretion theory. Krogh implied as much when he wrote his tepid evaluation of Haldane to Professor George Dreyer, a member of the Oxford selection committee (Schmidt-Nielsen 1995). "Even though I thoroughly disagree with Haldane on more than one point, as you know, I greatly respect his work and it would please me if he got it [the chair]." The coveted chair went to Sherrington, and Haldane withdrew to his own laboratory at home.

When the war was raging in Europe, Haldane wanted to help. Large numbers of British soldiers were being exposed to the dreadful effects of gas warfare, which had started with the German use of chlorine at the first battle of Ypres in 1915 and had progressed in 1917 to the use of the more deadly mustard gas. No one knew more than Haldane about the pulmonary effects of gases, but the government did not call upon him. Douglas, then a medical officer with the British military command in Flanders, frequently wrote to Haldane for advice on treatment of gassed soldiers. Sherrington involved him in animal experiments in Oxford on the effects of poison gases. But the official silence from the war office was deafening. Haldane did as much as he could, but as shown by his letter to Douglas of August 8, 1917, his correspondence had a plaintive tone. "All information of the anti-gas committee is [kept secret], so that I get no information except through people in France, or from what I can see for myself, or hear from scientific reports to the R. S. [Royal Society] Committee itself. I wish I could be of more help, but one is paralyzed by not knowing what is being done elsewhere." Haldane may even have thought his colleagues were avoiding him, for on August 18, 1917, he wrote, "I went up yesterday to the Royal Society Committee. There were a great many people there, but all seemed in a hurry to get away including Barcroft, whom I hadn't much chance of talking to." Perhaps his loyalty was questioned because his elder brother, Richard, who had been secretary of state for war, was suspected of having German sympathies. Or was his error over "oxygen secretion" a contributor?

In any event, within the space of a few months Haldane's most treasured concept had been rejected by the scientific community, he had been passed over by his university, and he had been ignored by his country in a time of great national crisis. He was an exceptionally strong and confident man, but he must have found this treatment dispiriting. He did no more work on oxygen secretion.

There is a parallel between the historical treatment of Oscar Wilde and Haldane. Both are now remembered by too many for the one mistake they refused to back away from, and both are remembered too little for their many great achievements. Wilde was imprisoned and destroyed for "posing as a sodomite"; Haldane lost the professorship he cherished, in part for believing too vehemently in his own experimental results regarding the secretion of oxygen. Of the two, Haldane has been dealt with more harshly. One hears, "Oh yes, Haldane, he's the one who got it wrong about oxygen secretion." This is a cruel misrepresentation of his achievements. The man who laid the very foundations of our understanding of the chemical control of breathing, including that at altitude, who made so many contributions to physiology, and who immeasurably improved working conditions and productivity in mines, factories, and under water deserves better than this.

We all, very reasonably, want to be judged by our best work. We deserve to be remembered for our greatest achievements. Haldane firmly laid the foundations for the understanding of altitude acclimatization by his new discoveries in 1911 on Pikes Peak, Colorado; let us not remember his expedition for its one pitfall. We owe it to him, and also to ourselves, to remember him for the phenomenal repertoire of seminal contributions that he made to the understanding of human physiology and to the well-being of humankind.

Appendix—
Some of Haldane's Other Scientific Contributions

As given in the following partial list, Haldane's scientific successes before and after Pikes Peak were indeed impressive. Haldane used his very sensitive apparatus to measure the amounts of gases in the air breathed out from the lung alveoli and to show for the first time the extraordinary sensitivity of the respiratory control system to carbon dioxide.[11] Previous workers had used complicated and unreliable techniques. They had, for example, estimated the normal composition of alveolar air from mixed expired gas, corrected by an inaccurate estimate of pulmonary dead space. And to test respiratory sensitivity they had given such high concentrations of carbon dioxide that the subjects were rendered nearly insensible. Haldane's exquisitely simple technique of obtaining alveolar air as the last part of an expired breath trapped near the mouth gave a pure sample that required no correction.

Although Haldane's gas analysis equipment requires patience and skill to use and can only analyze individual samples, it is still widely recognized as the most accurate way of establishing the composition of gases used for the calibration of modern equipment. He also developed the accurate method that depends on color for the measurement of hemoglobin concentration in blood (see fig. 3.3).

He developed a technique for measuring the total amount of oxygen in blood. He found that a chemical (ferricyanide) converted hemoglobin to an inactive form (methemoglobin) and drove off all the oxygen, which then could be measured. For many decades this was the principle for a simple, inexpensive, and accurate way of measuring the oxygen content of blood. It made clumsy, leak-prone vacuum pumps obsolete, and it required only one or two milliliter of blood. Knowledge of the precise oxygen content of many blood samples impressed upon him that "the colouring power of haemoglobin" is a function of oxygen saturation. The basic concept of today's oximeters, that oxygenation changes the color of blood, goes back to Haldane.

Using the instruments he had devised and his prodigious capacity for analysis, Haldane developed an equation that fit remarkably well the reaction of oxygen with hemoglobin (Douglas et al. 1912). It allowed accurate estimation of the oxygen level of a red cell at the midpoint between the beginning and end of the lung capillary. Haldane also correctly showed that at rest at sea level the red cells have acquired their full complement of oxygen in the lung after traversing only the first third of the capillary length (1912). He showed that as the venous blood is oxygenated in the lung, the hemoglobin becomes more acidic, which helps it unload carbon dioxide, a reaction known as the Haldane effect

(Christiansen et al. 1914). Haldane's development of new and powerful techniques, combined with a firm knowledge of physiology, brought new understanding to the control of breathing and to the transport of respiratory gases by hemoglobin.

In 1896 Haldane discovered the peculiar fact that bright light caused carbon monoxide to dissociate from hemoglobin. This turned out to be more than a methodological quirk, because in 1923 the principle was used to measure precisely the speeds with which carbon monoxide and oxygen react with hemoglobin (Hartridge and Roughton 1923) and, later, to examine the speed with which carbon monoxide combines with and poisons cytochrome oxidase (Warburg and Negelein 1929), which is essential for the burning of oxygen in the mitochondria. Unwittingly, Haldane had given biochemistry a near-perfect way of measuring the rate of important chemical reactions, using only transmitted and reflected light.

His use of carbon monoxide on Pikes Peak to measure the total amounts of hemoglobin and blood in the body had been based upon his earlier work (Douglas 1910), which showed that carefully calculated quantities of the gas rebreathed from a closed-circuit apparatus would not be harmful but would remain combined with hemoglobin for many minutes. Ironically, while his work with carbon monoxide improved the welfare of countless miners and led to numerous scientific advances, it brought him to grief on Pikes Peak where he thought he had proven the existence of "oxygen secretion." Carbon monoxide played immensely important roles, both positive and negative, in his life.

Normally the human lung is very effective in supplying oxygen to the blood and in removing carbon dioxide. But the lung worked poorly in soldiers gassed in the Great War of 1914–1918. Although Haldane was not officially consulted on this problem, he wrestled with it. Why should gassed soldiers have such poor arterial oxygenation even when breathing oxygen? He reasoned that part of the problem could be their pattern of rapid, shallow breathing. He found that when he placed a strap around the chest of a normal subject, breathing became rapid and shallow and the arterial oxygen became very low "in spite of the fact that alveolar [oxygen] is greater than normal." He likened the normal expansion of the lung upon inspiration to "the opening of a Japanese fan" with the lung segments near the diaphragm, which he correctly noted had the greatest ventilation, expanding first. He explained that when tidal volume is restricted by strapping, some lung segments became poorly ventilated, even though blood continued to perfuse them. In effect, the lung blood flow did not go to well-oxygenated lung regions. Haldane may have been the first to recognize the importance of matching ventilation to perfusion locally within the lung, although his contribution is rarely quoted. He stated that "the relationship between blood-supply and ventilation in individual groups of alveoli is not an even one," and he understood the need for "the distribution of air to individual lung alveoli to correspond exactly with the distribution of blood to them."

He also knew that because carbon dioxide was very soluble in plasma, it would be less affected by a mismatching than would oxygen with its complex binding to hemoglobin. Noting that a poor matching of ventilation and blood flow could profoundly lower the arterial oxygen level, he suggested that normally the lung might try to regulate blood vessels in such a way as to match local blood flow to ventilation. It was not until some decades later that the small arteries of the lung were found to perform such a function. Here again, Haldane was ahead of his time.

Notes

1. C. Gordon Douglas (1882–1963) was an English physician and Haldane's primary colleague in Oxford.
2. Yandell Henderson (1873–1944) was a professor of physiology from Yale University with interests in respiration and circulation. Apart from his participation in the Pikes Peak expedition he is probably best known for his work on medical shock.
3. Edward C. Schneider (1874–1954) had received his Ph.D. degree in physiology from Yale University and was a professor of biology at Colorado College in Colorado Springs. His laboratory served as the base of operation for the Pikes Peak expedition. His participation in the expedition certainly enhanced his scientific reputation, and he was a key consultant on aviation to the United States Army in World War I.
4. This chapter draws heavily on three main sources: (1) "The Regulation of Human Respiration," proceedings of the *J. S. Haldane Centenary Symposium* (Cunningham 1963), which contains Douglas's obituary of Haldane and other articles; (2) Haldane and Priestley's book *Respiration*, 2d ed. (1935); and (3) Douglas, Haldane, Henderson, and Schneider's report of their findings on Pikes Peak (1913). Some of the photographs are from the display in the physiology laboratory.
5. Sir Joseph Barcroft; see note 7, chap. 5.
6. Angelo Mosso (1847–1910) was the famous Italian high-altitude physiologist from Turin. He established in 1893 the Capanna Regina Margherita high-altitude laboratory at 14,960 feet on Monte Rosa.
7. "Battledore-and-shuttlecock," an ancient oriental game, which was the precursor of badminton.
8. August (1874–1949) and Marie (1874–1943) Krogh were a husband-and-wife team of physiologists from Copenhagen, Denmark, famous for their work in respiration and blood flow. August received the Nobel Prize in 1920 for his work on the capillary circulation.
9. Paul Bert, the famous French high-altitude physiologist, published in 1878 his *La Pression barométrique*, which showed that the symptoms observed at great altitudes result from the reduction in atmospheric oxygen with decreasing barometric pressure.
10. Sir Charles Sherrington (1857–1952) was the greatest neurophysiologist of his time. He had given the Silliman Lectures at Yale, published in 1906, an honor shared by some of England's most famous scientists—J. J. Thompson, Ernest Rutherford, Walter Nernst, Svante Arrhenius, and William Bateson. Sherrington's lecture was eleven years before Haldane's and seven years before being elected to

Oxford's Waynflete Chair of Physiology. Sherrington received the Nobel Prize in 1932 for his studies on the function of neurons.

11. Although Miescher-Rusch (1885) had concluded from his interpretation of the literature that carbon dioxide dominates the control of ventilation, Haldane gave the first quantitative description of this, showing in laboratory experiments that a rise of only 1.5 to 2 mm Hg in alveolar pressure of CO_2 doubles resting ventilation (Haldane and Priestley 1905). Haldane also showed that ventilation is essentially unaffected by alveolar PO_2 until it falls to below about 60 mm Hg. This at first suggested to Haldane that ventilation was almost always stimulated by CO_2, but he was soon to modify this view because he correctly deduced that in heavy exercise lactic acid released from working muscles stimulates the "respiratory centres" to increase breathing. This led him to propose that ventilation is determined by the total acidity of arterial blood, whether its source be respiratory carbon dioxide or a product of metabolism such as lactic acid. Later on Pikes Peak he further modified his ideas to include the important role of oxygen in ventilatory control.

3

MAJOR BREATHING IN MINERS

Mabel Purefoy FitzGerald, an Intrepid Scientist, Visits Colorado's High Mines

Robert W. Torrance, M.A., B.Sc., B.M., B.Ch., and John T. Reeves, M.D.

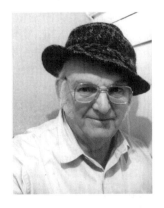

The late R. W. Torrance,[1] *left*, tells the story of Mabel FitzGerald of Oxford, who in 1911 was not to accompany the men to Pikes Peak but instead traveled alone to measure breathing in residents of the raucous mining camps around Colorado. In those Victorian times, how could an unmarried Englishwoman break the expected stereotype to make a fundamental scientific contribution in a society dominated by men? Her story is both fascinating and triumphant. As a student for more than two decades of FitzGerald's life, Torrance is qualified to write about her. He was a fellow of St. John's College, Oxford, and an eminent respiratory physiologist at Oxford University Laboratory of Physiology. Douglas, Haldane's associate and a member of the 1911 Pikes Peak expedition, was one of his mentors. Following FitzGerald's death, Torrance, more than anyone else, was responsible for the preservation of her papers, the source of much of this chapter, and her scientific equipment.

—THE EDITORS

Mabel Purefoy FitzGerald (fig. 3.1) is all but forgotten in the history of the study of human acclimatization to high altitude. This remarkable lady, born in Victorian England, single-handedly made a classic set of observations on the alterations in breathing in men and women living high in the Rocky Mountains of Colorado (1913, 1914). Traveling alone by narrow-gauge railroad, stagecoach, and horseback, this intrepid woman visited the brawling mining camps that dotted the mountains at various altitudes west of Colorado Springs in the early 1900s. It was a marvelous adventure in physiological research, which showed for the first time the large and sustained increase in breathing in men and women living at high altitude.

In spite of her pioneering accomplishments, FitzGerald has remained relatively unknown in scientific circles apart from her native England, probably because she worked in the shadow of John Scott Haldane, then the most distinguished of the English respiratory physiologists (chap. 2). When Haldane and his colleague, C. Gordon Douglas, planned their famous high-altitude expedition to Colorado in 1911, FitzGerald was included as a member of the research team. By prearrangement she did not participate in the well-known experiments on the summit of Pikes Peak. Rather she struck out on her own to study breathing in miners and other residents at various altitudes around Colorado. In a true sense she was a pioneering investigator. Like most of the other scientists in this book, and except for a visit to the lesser heights of the Appalachians, FitzGerald made only this single excursion into research at high altitude. Thereafter, her life moved in other directions. Indeed she would not be remembered at all if it were not for her extraordinary scientific adventure in Colorado, an adventure all the more remarkable because she was a woman performing research in a field that in those years was reserved for men. The time has come to revisit her life.

Mabel FitzGerald was an adventurer. She had first come to the United States in 1901, and in 1908 she traveled alone out west, going even to the Pacific Coast. Her postcard to Haldane told of her visit high in the Colorado mountains. "Oh I am having a glorious time. The Rockies are all that I anticipated. Today we have been riding up a lovely canyon, riding true western style, cross saddle. Washington a beautiful city. Chicago appalling. Denver good trip from there up Mt. McClellan, 14,000 ft. exquisite. Going on to New Mexico tonight."

She must have fallen in love with Colorado, because she returned in 1909. Having been joined by her favorite sister, Laura, who came over from England, she traveled around the western United States and Canada for three months. They visited Pikes Peak, which stands rather uniquely forward toward the east from the main body of the Rockies and close to the city of Colorado Springs. The sisters cleverly timed their visit to arrive at the mountaintop shortly before the sun rose magnificently over the plains to the east. They avoided the mountain sickness that waiting up there overnight would have given them.

But FitzGerald often spent part of the summer at home in Oxford, if she was not going off on some grand trip, for example, to the mountains of Colorado. She was in Oxford in the summer of 1910,

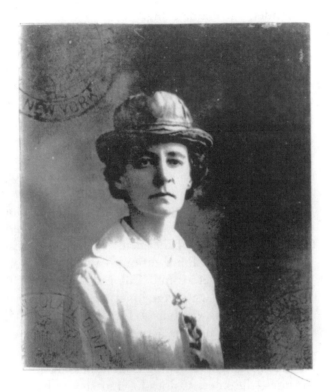

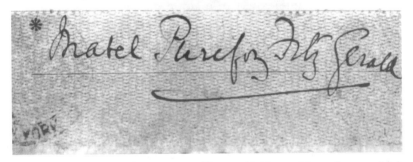

Fig. 3.1. Mabel Purefoy FitzGerald in a 1915 passport photo, which describes her as "aged 42, height 5 ft 5½ in tall, forehead medium, eyes blue, mouth medium, nose long, chin square, hair light brown." Courtesy Bodleian Library, Oxford.

when Haldane and his associate, Douglas, had just returned from the International Congress of Physiology in Vienna. There they had had a very long discussion of the physiology of high altitude with an American, Yandell Henderson. Haldane had said, "I want a nice comfortable, easily accessible, very high mountain with a fairly good hotel on top." Henderson replied, "Come to America next summer and we will spend a month or two on the top of Pikes Peak."

So that is how the famous expedition was conceived (Douglas et al. 1913). Among other things, Haldane wanted to know about the effect of sustained oxygen lack on breathing and the blood hemoglobin level in humans. The centerpiece of his plan was to describe how breathing changed after coming suddenly to Pikes Peak, and four men, Haldane and Douglas of Oxford, Henderson of Yale, and Schneider of Colorado College, would do this (see fig. 2.2). In addition Haldane wanted to know about breathing and hemoglobin in people who had long lived at altitude in Colorado, and this was where FitzGerald would come in. The team, then, would consist of the men, who were to be studied on the Peak as they developed acclimatization to altitude, and one woman, FitzGerald, who would travel around Colorado studying full acclimatization in men and women who were longtime residents at the various altitudes. Although she was visiting Oxford that summer, there is no record showing whether or not she actually joined in those discussions, but it is difficult to believe she did not. She had the expertise needed for measurements of breathing and hemoglobin in persons in a steady state at various altitudes, she knew Colorado, and she had even visited the summit of Pikes Peak, on which the observations were to be made.

FitzGerald had been working for some years with Haldane in his laboratory. She had wanted to enter the university, but in those years Oxford did not admit women, so she came to work for Haldane as a technician. She became expert in making measurements on breathing, for example, measuring levels of carbon dioxide in air trapped at the end of an expiration. She thus obtained carbon dioxide levels in air from the alveoli, which are the air sacs deep in the lung. Haldane and Priestley had published the technique in 1905 and knew that the carbon dioxide level closely related to the amount of air breathed. When breathing increases, carbon dioxide (which is blown off) decreases. And when breathing decreases, carbon dioxide (which is retained) increases. FitzGerald mastered the demanding, but accurate, Haldane apparatus for these measurements of carbon dioxide in alveolar air.

She was an expert at making surveys of breathing, and she loved doing it. She had started by making measurements in herself, which she did daily over more than two years. And she made frequent measurements in Haldane and in his colleague, Priestley. Because the carbon dioxide level remained remarkably constant at rest, it could determine the amount of air breathed, which also remained fairly constant at rest. And following a long bicycle ride, FitzGerald's carbon dioxide level was the same as at rest. Apparently the amount of air breathed was closely matched to the amount of energy the body used, and Haldane felt the level of carbon dioxide was the likely regulator. FitzGerald published this paper, with Haldane, in 1905. Respiratory physiologists are still trying to understand how the body manages precise matching of ventilation to metabolic requirements.

The paper also included a careful and thorough investigation of breathing in twenty-seven men, thirty-two women, sixteen boys, and eleven girls in Oxford. The children had come from the Dragon School and were great fun; they included Haldane's son Jack. FitzGerald had also studied Haldane's brilliant daughter, who was to become the prolific and eccentric novelist Naomi Mitchison. Among the adults she had studied were her own sisters and Haldane's brother, later to become the lord chancellor of England. She found that women and children breathed more than men.

She was right. As men grow older, they are often notoriously poor breathers. It is men, not women or children, who most often are "lazy breathers" and thus at risk for breathing disorders during sleep, when they become overweight, when they develop emphysema, or when they have lived for many decades at high altitude. Indeed, the sex hormones have important influences on breathing; the female hormone progesterone is a powerful stimulant. Pregnant women are awash in progesterone, which largely accounts for their high breathing rates (chap. 6). On the other hand, the male hormone testosterone inhibits breathing. In fact, sometimes men who are "lazy breathers" are treated with progesterone to make them breathe better. All of these concepts have their roots in FitzGerald's 1905 paper.

She did a remarkable survey of breathing in patients at the Radcliffe Infirmary in Oxford in 1910. At that time, especially among women fourteen to twenty years of age who worked as domestic servants, anemia was very common because they could not afford to eat the protein and iron required to replace those lost in menstrual blood. The extreme anemia and fatigue led to hospital admissions for weeks of treatment with tablets containing iron. Although these young women had hemoglobin levels as low as one-fourth the normal value, their lungs were healthy. In their arterial blood each red blood cell carried its full complement of oxygen and was fully saturated, but with so few red cells, the total amount of oxygen in the blood was much reduced.

Did the profound anemia affect their breathing and would their breathing change as the anemia improved? The patients presented an opportunity to learn, in people with healthy lungs, how breathing was controlled, that is, whether either the level of oxygen saturation in the blood or the total amount of oxygen was important. From September 1905 to March 1906, FitzGerald made repeated measurements in nineteen anemic women as they recovered in the hospital. Her findings showed their breathing at rest remained surprisingly normal even when they were severely anemic. Little or no change occurred on recovery, and she noted that the amount of hemoglobin or the number of red blood cells did not seem to affect breathing at rest.

Fortunately she also studied a sixteen-year-old girl with congenital heart disease who had a blue color, with low saturation of oxygen in her blood, which caused very high hemoglobin concentrations and high red blood cell counts. The girl probably had tetralogy of Fallot, in which an obstruction at the outlet of the right ventricle and a hole in the ventricular septum caused some of the venous blood to bypass the lung and go directly into the systemic circulation. This would have caused her blue color. FitzGerald found the girl had markedly increased breathing and attributed it to a low arterial oxygen saturation. In this girl, her breathing was controlled by the low oxygen saturation and not by the hemoglobin level. FitzGerald's conclusions even anticipated her findings in Colorado, for she speculated on what might happen at high altitude: breathing is increased "owing to the incomplete saturation of the arterial blood with oxygen."

With all this experience she was the perfect person to join the expedition to Colorado. She even may have suggested they include a scientist from Colorado College in the expedition. On March 24, 1911, in response to her letter, Haldane replied, "A base of operations at Colorado Springs will be an enormous help." Then in May, Haldane wrote her that Edward C. Schneider, a professor of biology at Colorado College, would join the expedition. But whether FitzGerald herself could come to Colorado was in doubt, and it was a question of money. She was counting on rental income from the house in Oxford. Yale University and a grant to Haldane from the Royal Society provided for her rail transport, but in those days a physiologist was a gentleman who was supposed to pay his own living expenses. She had worried Haldane at the outset, because she was not able to commit to the expedition until two weeks before Haldane sailed for America, but she proved worth waiting for because, after all, she was the great surveyor of breathing and hemoglobin in populations.

Douglas and Haldane set off for Colorado on June 24, 1911, and the whole team, including FitzGerald, met on July 7 in Colorado Springs.

Douglas and Haldane, with ten cases of scientific equipment, had traveled first by sea and then to Colorado by train. Henderson traveled from New Haven, Connecticut. Schneider had returned to Colorado Springs from Yale, where he had visited Henderson to learn techniques of respiratory physiology. Previously, Schneider had only measured a few blood pressures at altitude. Later, in the war of 1914–1918, his 1911 work on Pikes Peak would make him a valuable scientist for the United States Air Force, for it gave him experience in the effects on man of acute and maintained exposure to low-oxygen environments. The five scientists worked together at Colorado College from July 8 through 12, setting up their apparatus and making preliminary observations. Then the men went off to the top of Pikes Peak by cog railway to spend five weeks in the summit house, studying in themselves the changes of acclimatization to altitude.

At first, FitzGerald continued in Colorado Springs and completed her observations for the height of 6,000 feet. Then she set off on her travels around Colorado. We do not know all those who helped plan the travels, but she thanked President Slocum of Colorado College; Mr. Peck, president of Portland Mine; Mr. S. A. Ionides of Denver; and a Mr. G. B. Young. A family friend, Heneage Griffin, an Englishman and Oxford graduate who had once owned mines in Colorado, also may have advised her. In addition Gerald Webb,[2] a prominent Colorado Springs physician, would have been of great help, for he had remained close to the Haldane expedition from the outset and he counted white blood cells in the men while they were on the summit.

FitzGerald said that "Colorado proved eminently suitable" for her purpose, because she wanted to make observations at various altitudes between Denver and the high mines. Measurements were made in large towns—Denver (5,100 feet) and Colorado Springs (6,000 feet); small towns in the mining areas—Ridgway, Ouray, and Telluride; and then the highest mines where the miners lived and worked—Portland, Camp Bird, Tom Boy, and Lewis Mines.[3] She also included Altman, "a declining mining camp which still boasts its position as the highest incorporated town in America."

She went to the towns in order of accessibility, not of increasing altitude. When she had finished in Colorado Springs on July 16, she visited the men on the Peak (see fig. 2.2) for a few hours before moving west behind the Peak to the Cripple Creek area. At the Portland Mine, a Dr. Jones was very helpful to her, and he later reported that he had greatly enjoyed her visit. She also studied men and women around Altman and then moved north to work in Denver, but she called in on the men on the Peak again for the second time as she passed by on July

30. By this time she had acclimatized in Altman, and she had no trouble with mountain sickness on the Peak as had previously occurred. She then went about three hundred miles west to Ouray and on to Telluride for the highest mines. By August 28 she had returned to Colorado Springs, but then she went off on a purely sightseeing trip into Utah and Salt Lake City. She was back in New York to see Douglas and Haldane before they set sail for England on September 9.

FitzGerald traveled mostly by rail, but occasionally on foot, on horseback, or by stagecoach. These journeys through "very wild and high mountains" were some of the things she greatly enjoyed. She loved riding in the western fashion, cross saddle, and not the ladylike English sidesaddle. By 1911 Colorado was laced with railroads, which had been built to serve the gold and silver mines and the growing populations associated with the mining industry. Denver could easily be reached from Colorado Springs over the Santa Fe or the Denver & Rio Grande Railroad. For the other destinations, she described her journey and her impressions:

> The Cripple Creek district, an open mountain country, formerly a cattle range, is between 50 and 60 miles by rail from Colorado Springs and looks out on the west side of Pikes Peak. In this district, Victor formed the base and the places visited from there, the Portland Mine and Mill (altitude 10,900 and 10,300 feet, respectively) and Altman (altitude 10,870 feet) were reached by an electric railway or on foot. The Ouray district situated in the southwestern part of the State, in the midst of very wild and mountainous country, was reached through the Grand Canyon of the Arkansas River [fig. 3.2] over the Marshall Pass, crossing the Continental Divide at a height of 10,856 feet, thence through the Black Canyon of the Gunnison and into the valley of the Uncompahgré River in which were situated two of the selected centres for work, the towns of Ridgway (altitude 6,990 feet) and Ouray (altitude 7,780 feet). Ridgway is in an open part of the valley, though in the neighborhood of Mount Uncompahgré (altitude 14,420 feet). Ouray, one of the oldest of the Colorado mining camps, is situated in a basin, and, to all appearance, completely walled in by rugged mountain ranges, varying in height from 10,000 to 13,500 feet (Whitehouse Mountain, Hayden Mountain, etc.)
>
> The Camp Bird Mill (altitude 9,500 feet), with its colony of miners, shut in at the head of a gulch, was reached from Ouray by mountain "stage." From the Mill up to the Camp Bird Mine (altitude 11,300 feet), about 2,000 feet above it and a distance of about 2 miles, the journey was made on horseback, while the gas analysis apparatus and other equipment reached the same destination by means of an aerial tramway used for the transportation of ore and the conveyance of supplies to the mine. Round the mine, the country is bleak and Mount

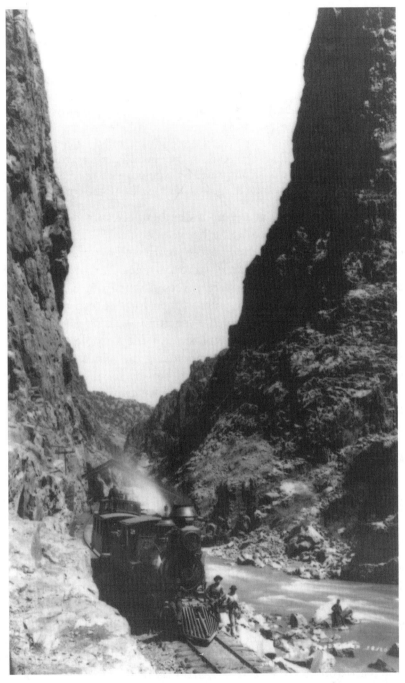

Fig. 3.2. The famous hanging bridge, a regular tourist stop on the narrow-gauge railroad through the Grand Canyon of the Arkansas (later called the Royal Gorge). FitzGerald loved this train trip through "wild and high mountains." Photograph by William Henry Jackson, ca 1911. Courtesy Colorado Historical Society.

Sueffles [sic] (altitude 14,158 feet) is close by. The condition of the
trail, owing to deep snow, prevented an approach on horseback from
the Camp Bird Mine to the high mines in the neighborhood of Telluride, which place had then to be reached, with loss of valuable time,
by the Rio Grande Southern Railway from Ridgway. Observations
were made at Telluride (altitude 8,770 feet), situated in the St. Miguel
Valley amidst very wild and high mountains, and thence at two
neighboring mines, the Tom Boy (altitude 11,500 feet), a few miles to
the north-east accessible by a good wagon road, and the Lewis
(altitude 12,500 feet) several miles by trail in another direction,
reached on horseback, accompanied by a guide, with the gas analysis
apparatus and equipment strapped to our saddles. (FitzGerald 1913)

Fortunately violence at the mines had largely subsided by 1911. In
Telluride in 1901 a pitched battle between some 250 armed union and
nonunion miners had resulted in the death and wounding of several
men, and the nonunion "scabs" were marched out of the county. In
1904 at Tom Boy the tables were reversed when one hundred armed
deputies rounded up some sixty union men for a forced midnight train
ride out of town. At Altman in 1903 the gun battles involved more than
a thousand men. In 1904, an explosion at the Cripple Creek railway
station killed thirteen nonunion men, closing the mines and even all the
saloons. The Colorado National Guard had been called in to maintain
order, and dozens of men, considered to be troublemakers, were de-
ported by rail to Kansas and New Mexico. But in the relatively tranquil
year of 1911, FitzGerald was received royally as a distinguished visitor
from Oxford: the leading citizens of the mining camps were her subjects, and she made the local news.

She enjoyed the best hospitality available and was featured on the
front page of the *Ouray Plaindealer* on August 11, 1911, as a "member
of a famous scientific expedition on a mission of vital importance." The
article notes that she "took the opportunity of thanking Dr. Rowan in
his capacity not only as mayor . . . but as . . . the oldest physician in the
town, for the many courtesies shown her." She was a celebrity, and she
reveled in it. In a large town she might set up to make measurements in
some grand office of a mining engineer and work with local professional people and students as her subjects, but out in the remote wild
areas she lived with the miners and the managers, and they, along with
their families, were her subjects. The Coloradans, both miners and pro-
fessionals, readily took to this lady from Oxford, and she had no difficulty persuading them to be subjects for her experiments.

Usually she studied groups of ten men, but the numbers were smaller
for women. Her standards for accepting someone as a subject were

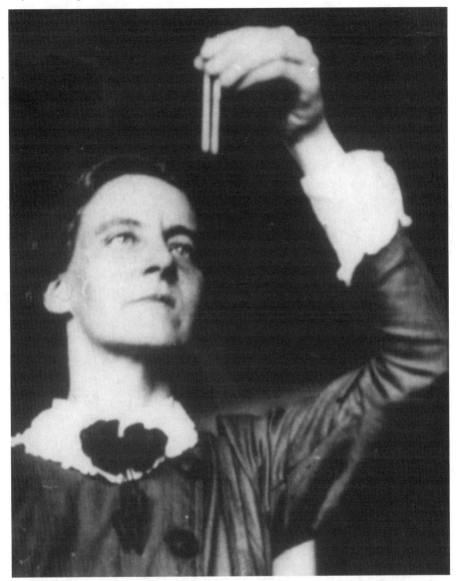

Fig. 3.3. *Mabel FitzGerald, measuring the hemoglobin in the blood by diluting a sample of blood in one of two tubes until it matches the color of the standard in the other tube. Reprinted from* Colorado Springs Herald Telegraph, *July 8, 1911.*

strict: one had to have lived at altitude for a year and at exactly the same height for the six weeks before being studied. She measured two things of interest, the amount of hemoglobin in the blood and the carbon dioxide in the alveolar air from the lungs. For the first she diluted a

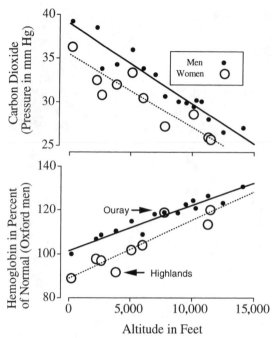

Fig. 3.4. Measurements made by Mabel FitzGerald. Top, alveolar carbon dioxide levels (measured as pressure) fall with increasing altitude in both men and women. Bottom, hemoglobin concentrations increase (measured as percent of normal) with increasing altitude in both men and women. Haldane complained of the levels found in the women of Highlands, North Carolina, and Ouray, Colorado, which are indicated by arrows. Drawn from data of Fitz-Gerald, 1913, 1914.

small sample of blood from a pricked finger until its color matched a standard (fig. 3.3). For the carbon dioxide she drew a sample of the subject's air after a full expiration, thus getting the gas that had been deep within the lungs. Using her gas analyzing apparatus, she measured how much the gas volume was reduced by absorbing the carbon dioxide, and from this and the barometric pressure she calculated her results. She carried in her "explorers pack" a simple aneroid barometer, which she calibrated with barometric pressures from meteorological stations in Denver and Colorado Springs and by comparison with other official readings for the district. All her published observations were related to these barometric pressures and not to the reported altitudes of the towns and mines, which differ slightly from more recent measurements. Her results show the fall in carbon dioxide and the rise in hemoglobin as one ascends from sea level (fig. 3.4).

So what were her scientific contributions in Colorado? Simply put, over the long term, even for all of life, it is oxygen, and not carbon dioxide, that overwhelmingly determines how much we breathe. Further, this control by oxygen level is sensitive to slight changes in altitude of residence and holds true over the whole range of altitudes at which human populations live. Haldane's previous ideas of the importance of carbon dioxide were not completely wrong. Carbon dioxide is the key regulator for the short term, minutes and hours. But when one goes to stay at high altitude, the body increases breathing to defend its oxygen supply, and over several days carbon dioxide is set to a new and lower level, where it remains. Haldane and his colleagues on Pikes Peak showed for one altitude, 14,110 feet, that the time required for the full resetting to occur was about one or two weeks. But it was FitzGerald who showed the sensitive, lasting, and overwhelming role for oxygen in breathing. She revolutionized our ideas of how breathing is controlled lifelong.

These are the measurements for which we now remember her. The plan and the measurements themselves may seem simple enough, but nothing better has been done since on her two variables for the range of altitudes she studied. Indeed few, if any, other variables have been measured systematically with the thoroughness and care with which she measured carbon dioxide at the various altitudes. At all altitudes, women had lower carbon dioxide levels than men because they breathed more (fig. 3.4), and their hemoglobin levels were lower than in men. These were the first such gender-related observations ever reported for altitude-acclimatized persons, and they have withstood the test of time. Furthermore, subsequent generations of mountain climbers have extended the lines drawn through her measurements to estimate how much air will be breathed and what the level of arterial oxygen might be in acclimatized persons going to great heights.

Afterward Haldane told FitzGerald, "Your work has been much more adventurous than ours!" But her work had involved a sort of travel she delighted in, and it had proceeded exactly as had been planned, except when snow on a pass blocked the trail.

When Douglas and Haldane got back to Oxford, the men proceeded rapidly with writing up their joint paper on the work on the Peak, but Haldane had to beg FitzGerald for a copy of her paper. He even begged for her tables of results, offering to do the paper himself. But life in New York had become busy. Because in America she could obtain the education that Oxford had denied her, she again thought of becoming a physician. To apply to medical school she needed a degree, and for this she entered New York University.

The premedical studies were time-consuming. An essay of hers, written in New York City, discusses the conditions for a police force to be honest. And all of the work did not go easily, for there were some examinations that really stuck. She finished American history in 24 hours and physics in 28 hours, but algebra took 173 hours. Haldane remarked: "I heard that you got ploughed [failed] in algebra and sincerely sympathize. I suffered much from examiners myself and was ploughed in physiology besides other similar experiences."

Her social life may also have interfered with the writing-up of her results from Colorado. She had developed a large circle of friends and acquaintances throughout the United States and especially in the East. In summer her practice was to escape the heat of New York City by going to the mountains or to fashionable Rhode Island estates. One of her friends, Richard Winning, a Harvard man and a lawyer on Wall Street, was a member of a family from Pojac Point, Rhode Island, and he had known her since 1901. Winning and Eleanor Roosevelt were both interested in the National Self Government Committee, and they may have drawn her in, for she wrote her sisters: "Dearest Girls, I lunched with Mrs. Franklin Roosevelt last Sunday, the senator's wife . . . she asked me to stay at Hyde Park, their country place up the Hudson, so you see I am being taken up by the 400! and today Mrs. Forbes asked me to dine" (Torrance, p.c.).

Although Pikes Peak may have been temporarily pushed aside, her paper came out on February 28, 1913, in the prestigious Philosophical Transactions of the Royal Society of London. As a result of her work in Colorado, Yandell Henderson, who was always her strong supporter, recommended her for membership in the American Physiology Society, and she was elected in 1913 as its second woman member.

After Colorado, but before she returned home to England in 1915 to help there during the Great War, FitzGerald's regular base was in New York City. Haldane contacted her there to ask that she study subjects acclimatized to lesser heights than those studied in Colorado. So in the summer of 1913 she studied subjects between 2,000 and 4,000 feet in the Appalachians of North Carolina. She did this as in Colorado, but now she had her own gas analysis apparatus and no longer suffered from the fickleness of the United States Customs Service, which had insisted on Haldane taking his apparatus back to Oxford. Her two sets of observations on the alveolar gases, those made in 1911 and in 1913, are consolidated in the graphs of the second paper and they fit together well (fig. 3.4), leading her to write of the combined data: "The results of the present investigation (for altitudes up to 3,850 feet) are in accord with those obtained with persons acclimatized at altitudes of 5,000 to 14,000 feet, and support the conclusion previously published that the lowering [of carbon dioxide] is in direct proportion to the diminution of the barometric pressure."

The combined results provided the foundation for our concepts of the control of breathing in general and ventilatory acclimatization to altitude in particular. Haldane would no longer believe lactic acidosis drove the increased breathing on arrival at altitude (chap. 2). Nor would breathing return in a few days to the sea-level norm for those who continued to live at altitude. The progressive increase in ventilation for several days after arrival ruled out arterial lactate as a factor. As a result of FitzGerald's work the message became clear. Breathing is exquisitely sensitive to changes in the amount of oxygen in the atmosphere. Even a small increase in the height of residence above sea level causes a sustained increase in breathing.

There were some minor details that didn't fit as well as Haldane would have liked (fig. 3.4). He commented about the hemoglobin measurements: "They make beautiful graphic representations except for the ladies of Ouray who for some reason have too much hemoglobin and ought never to have been born." Later he commented, "The women of Highlands [North Carolina] are, like the ladies of Ouray, a disgrace to physiology as regards their hemoglobin. It was lucky that the men's hemoglobin played up [behaved]."

All those in Ouray who volunteered to be subjects were the leading citizens of the community, including the venerable town physician, Mayor Rowan. The "ladies of Ouray" who were a "disgrace to physiology" and "ought never to have been born" had been named in the *Ouray Plaindealer* of August 11. One of the women listed, Mrs. E. C. Weatherly, was the wife of a distinguished 1878 graduate of Brasenose College, Oxford. Weatherly himself was also a subject in FitzGerald's studies, was the author of the *Plaindealer* article, and was a regular contributor to the newspaper. The ladies were the cream of Ouray society, and they certainly would not have been appreciative of Haldane's remarks, had they known. But in his famous 1916 Silliman Lecture at Yale (1917), Haldane included their data, and he presented in a single figure all of the results in both men and women, for both alveolar gases and hemoglobin.

Who was this adventurer who made scientific history in the high Colorado altitudes? Born in 1872, FitzGerald was brought up in England in the ways of her time as a member of a landowning family, one of the landed gentry, who lived in the country fairly near to London. The gentry had no hereditary title, but until only a short time before her birth they had exercised power in their villages. In her day they were candidates for membership on the local county council, and they tended to get elected to it. They did not have to own much land to belong to the gentry; 300 acres would do. Some of them were very rich, but others were far from that. The fortunate man of a generation of the family held the land; the others went into the armed services or into the established church or practiced law. They talked to the aristocracy and might marry into it, but they rejected the commercial middle class.

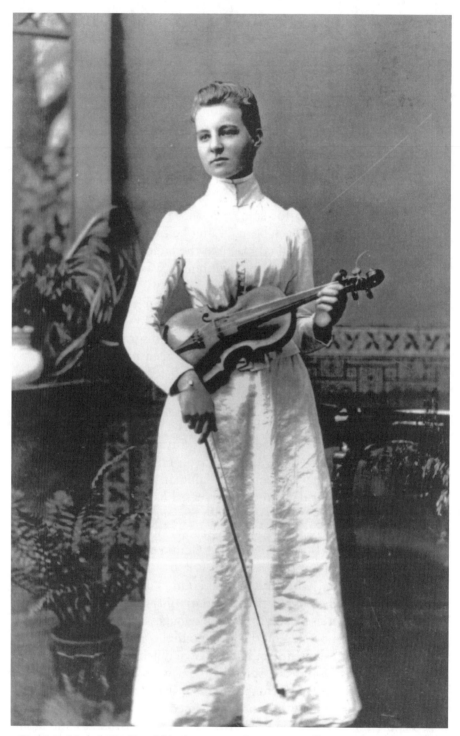

Fig. 3.5. Mabel FitzGerald in her teens. Courtesy Bodleian Library, Oxford.

FitzGerald came from a family that owned two lots of land, each about fifty miles west of London. Her mother was a parson's daughter, and her father had at first been in the military. He then became a manager of the family land; they rang the bells of the village church to celebrate his birthday. FitzGerald had an elder brother, who had joined the navy in his early teens and had trained with the future King George V. Her younger brother had received a conventional education at a public school and then read science at Oxford. He taught at Wellington, a great school, and then went into the church. She adored him for his science.

For her first twenty-two years FitzGerald lived with her parents in Preston Candover near to Basingstoke and about five miles from Steventon, where Jane Austen had been born, and both Jane Austen and Mabel FitzGerald grew up amongst the same class of landed gentry. Jane Austen had written of this landed gentry in her novels one hundred years earlier. Like the five Bennet daughters in Austen's *Pride and Prejudice*, there were five daughters in the FitzGerald family, but none of the FitzGerald five ever got married. For marriage young women depended on great beauty or a good dowry, which the FitzGerald sisters did not possess. In Victorian England life for women was less exciting and held fewer opportunities than for men. Girls were educated at home. For activities they walked, cycled, painted, acted in amateur theatricals, and made music. Mabel, the youngest of the five daughters, studied French and once spent a holiday in Le Havre. She also played the violin (fig. 3.5). So that was FitzGerald's early life: the life of an unmarried country lady who was dependent on her parents.

This picture of stability changed abruptly early in 1895. Her mother was operated on for a tumor by a surgeon in London. While she was recovering there, her father, who was then running for election to the local council, caught pneumonia and died. Her mother returned home, but soon she too died. The children put a window in the south aisle of the church at Preston Candover to commemorate them. As was the custom, the house and land were inherited by the elder, naval brother. The five girls immediately went to live with their grandmother at Shalstone about twenty miles north of Oxford. There in the garden at Shalstone FitzGerald wrote in her diary about reading the classical physiology text of Thomas H. Huxley.[4] She began to attend lectures on health, and she made the acquaintance of the local doctor, Dr. D'eath, "a real good friend to me."

What should she do with her life, now being much less tied down by her family? She loved science and was inclined toward a career in medicine. Also, a new and optimistic medical age had dawned. With the scientific discoveries of the prior decade, bacteria were known as the cause of tuberculosis and many other dread diseases of the day. Dr. D'eath, who was also an officer of health, was well informed about the new and exciting findings in bacteriology. He encouraged her to study in the medical field. At Shalstone in early 1896 she seems to have decided on a career in laboratory medical science. So, when she was in her early twenties, she had already decided to revolt against the norm in her social class at the time, namely, the unfulfilling life of an unmarried woman.

The deaths of the parents appear to have liberated the children. Both of the sons soon married, and the five daughters began looking for a house in Oxford. Perhaps they chose Oxford for its location between Shalston and Preston Candover; besides life in a university town would be more interesting than in a rural setting. In 1896 the five FitzGerald sisters moved to Oxford and bought a house just north of the University Science Laboratory and within easy walking distance of it across University Parks. The house, built in 1877, is still there at 12 Crick Road. It was part of the red-brick development of Oxford toward the north, started in the second half of the nineteenth century and now famous as North Oxford. In their day it was thought of as a rather small house, but there were five bedrooms and three baths, arranged on three floors, so the sisters fitted nicely into it. It was their base for the rest of their lives; for Mabel FitzGerald that was from 1896 to 1973.

FitzGerald had long been interested in the function of the human body. She had read Huxley and gone to lectures in nursing, physiology, and other medical sciences, and now she had a good chance in Oxford of getting into this world of science more fully. Her friend Dr. D'eath had advised her to take a course such as physiology before she started research. The university did not officially admit women to study physiology for medicine, but the laboratory let her attend classes there informally from 1896 to 1899. She made top grades in the examinations, but they did not count toward a degree because as a woman she could not be officially enrolled.

The histologist Gustav Mann was her first mentor in the laboratory, and she helped him with his teaching and with getting his book on histological technique ready for the press. Somehow during this time she was able to do independent research; a paper of hers on the spinal cord showed her as the only author. During this period she also went to lectures in pathology and on topics other than physiology. It is not known whether she worked in the laboratory as a lady of independent means, living on her inheritance, or whether she was employed as Gustav

Mann's assistant and received an income, which would have been welcome in this household of unmarried sisters. She also spent short periods on pathological subjects in Cambridge and in Denmark with her Danish friend Georges Dreyer, who was shortly to become professor of pathology in Oxford. She had made his acquaintance when he was in Oxford working with Burdon Sanderson, Haldane's uncle, then the professor of physiology. Already in the early 1900s she had herself set up and going in science.

This early background in science gave FitzGerald a good basis for her work with Haldane. Oddly she and Haldane lived next door to one another on Crick Road during her first few years in Oxford, but Haldane asserts that they did not know one another until she had become active in physiology. By then he had moved away from Crick Road. Thus he did not draw her into physiology, though he did get her into the field of respiration, where she did her best-known work. But respiration was far from the only subject she worked upon. With some of the world's most distinguished scientists she performed research at a very high level and on a wide range of medical subjects. Although here we focus on her work on altitude, her papers on gastric secretion (1910b, 1910–1911b) were extremely well done, and she worked in infectious diseases (1907, 1908, 1910–1911a) and other subjects in pathology. She was interested in most of the laboratory work of her day in medicine but, being a woman, she could not enter Oxford to get a degree.

In 1905 Sir William Osler had become the Regius Professor of Medicine in Oxford,[5] and it was he who had welcomed her to study his patients in the Radcliffe infirmary. She was charmed by Sir William and his wife, and he interested her in old medical books and helped with her career. He encouraged her to apply for a Rockefeller Fellowship, and she got it. At the very end of 1907 she set sail for the United States. In mid-Atlantic she was charmed by flowers from him, just as he and Mrs. Osler had been charmed a year or two earlier by flowers from her. Compared to Osler, with his warm personality, Haldane was a pure intellectual.

FitzGerald arrived in New York City very early in January 1908 and took up her fellowship at the Rockefeller Institute. She lived in an apartment at 416 East Sixty-fifth Street to the east of the south end of Central Park. At first she worked in bacteriology with Noguchi,[6] and her work is described in a paper on sporulation in bacilli (1910–1911a). Flexner was head of the Institute,[7] but she seems not to have got on well with him, possibly because she was so independent. In addition, there may have been some misunderstanding about whether she would definitely return from the fellowship in the United States to work with the new professor of pathology, her friend Georges Dreyer. In any event she gladly left New York after six months and, following a tour of the western United States, went to work on secretion of gastric acid with Macallum in Toronto.[8]

She felt welcomed by Macallum and produced results so quickly in her new subject that they were reported by Macallum at the Baltimore meeting of the American Physiological Society in December of 1908. The men from Rockefeller who attended the meeting congratulated her, except for Flexner, who seemed embarrassed by her success since leaving Rockefeller. Her paper on gastric secretion of acid appeared in the Proceedings of the Royal Society of London with her again as the sole author (1910–1911b).

By 1914 FitzGerald had worked in the United States or Canada for some five years. How did she manage? Initially she was supported by her grant from the Rockefeller Institute. Yale University paid her for helping Yandell Henderson with experiments on respiration. Probably on Henderson's recommendation, she worked for the American Navy Ventilation Commission, and a letter from Haldane doubted whether she was being paid enough. She probably also worked in a hospital as a clinical pathologist, for that was the profession listed on her passport when she left the United States for Edinburgh in 1915. Also, she may have taught, as she is referred to as "representing a scientific school" in a press description of the Pikes Peak team. She may have brought some of her own money from England. But despite these uncertainties, letters to her in New York were always addressed to 416 East Sixty-fifth Street near to Central Park. Although she was not rich, she was much better off than O'Henry's shop girls living across New York City in Brickdust Row on a total of six dollars per week. Not only did FitzGerald manage to live in some comfort, but also she paid for her own premedical studies at New York University.

After her two papers reporting altitude results from Colorado and from North Carolina, she published no other research from her time in the United States. By now, war was raging in Europe. Survival of her country was at stake, and her laboratory skills as a clinical pathologist were sorely needed. The call came from Professor Ritchie in Edinburgh, who had known her when he was professor of pathology in Oxford. He asked her to join the pathology laboratory in Edinburgh, where Lorrain Smith, a pupil of Haldane's, was professor. Not only could she help in this crisis, but there was also the opportunity of doing research there. Giving up her cherished idea of medical school, she accepted, returning to the United Kingdom in early 1915. She brought her gas analysis apparatus back with her; it is now on display in the Oxford Laboratory of

Physiology and is still labeled "Highlands Sanatorium" and "White Star Line."

She stood in for a Dr. Logan, who had gone off to the war, and the history of clinical bacteriology in Edinburgh reports him as being replaced by "a Miss FitzGerald." She seems now to be forgotten there; it has been the physicians who were remembered, and she had no degree at all, let alone a medical one. In Edinburgh, 54a George Square now replaced 416 East Sixty-fifth Street, New York City, as her outstation from 12 Crick Road in Oxford, where three of her sisters remained. The eldest, Geraldine, had died in 1900. The three remaining sisters had not trained for a profession and did various jobs in the war such as nursing and book mending in the Bodleian Library. Mary was classified as being involved in "domestic duties." In contrast to Mabel's life, their lives were far from exciting, and one of them wondered, "What use am I? Why hang around?"

Because FitzGerald was so capable in the laboratory, she was soon sought after. The Lister Institute in London asked her to set up for them a collection of type cultures of bacteria. Edinburgh physicians consulted her about their patients with infections. When Haldane went to the United States in 1916 to give his Silliman Lectures at Yale, she even had him pick up some glass pipettes for her laboratory. She soon built up a position for herself in the medical circles of Edinburgh. Though she had no degree, she even became an official lecturer in the Second Royal Colleges' Medical School of Edinburgh after being examined by the Edinburgh College of Physicians. In those years women were taught in the lesser school. Some of her lecture notes remain. Being a woman, it was particularly remarkable that she also became an extracurricular examiner in the larger university medical school for men.

Dr. Logan came back from the war and took up his old job. Again, as she had done in New York, FitzGerald seems to have accumulated a variety of things to do. Teaching and practicing laboratory medicine somewhere near Edinburgh could have been her reason for retaining her base in George Square. She collected and sold rare old medical books. Osler had interested her in them soon after he came to Oxford in 1905, and a city like Edinburgh, with its long history of medical scholarship, was a good place to find old books. Osler's biographer, H. W. Cushing, received her list of books and bought from her.[9] For her, old medical books were a commercial operation. She also sought out books for the Osler Library after Osler had died in 1919, and the library was being prepared by Osler's widow and a nephew to be moved to Montreal.

FitzGerald was a close friend of Dr. J. J. Graham Brown (1853–1925), a distinguished Edinburgh clinical teacher, who had recently been

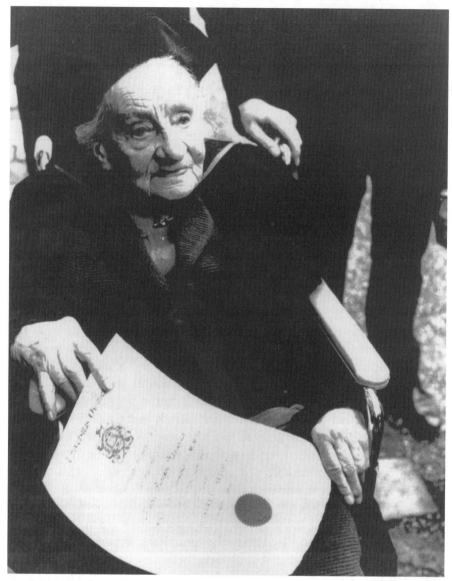

Fig. 3.6. Mabel FitzGerald, at age 101, with her honorary Master of Arts degree
from Oxford University, December 1972. From the Oxford Mail, December 14,
1972. Reprinted, by permission, from the Oxford Mail.

president of the Edinburgh College of Physicians. In 1885 the Royal
Society of Medicine had sent him to study the cholera epidemic in Spain.
Her responsibilities for the bacteriological aspects of patients would

have brought her into contact with such a physician, and he may well have helped her obtain her lectureships.

Shortly before World War II, when she was about sixty-five, FitzGerald gave up Edinburgh and returned to Oxford to 12 Crick Road. She settled into retirement in North Oxford, where she was known by her neighbors, particularly Roger Elliott, the theoretical physicist of St. John's College, and his wife, Olga. But oddly the physiology laboratory, where Douglas still worked, had no idea where she was. In 1961 Dan Cunningham, a member of the laboratory, was organizing the celebration of the Haldane centenary, and while looking up a number in the Oxford telephone directory came by chance upon the name Mabel P. FitzGerald. She was still living on 12 Crick Road, across University Parks to the north and less than half a mile away. She was eighty-eight and was the only one of the sisters remaining. She actually came to a part of the Haldane celebrations.

FitzGerald was still living at 12 Crick Road when she reached the age of one hundred in 1972. Her life took off once more, and she again became a celebrity, as reported by her niece, Mrs. Brian Purefoy, to Dr. Bruce Dill (see chap. 5) of the American Physiological Society:

> The famous birthday on August 3rd was a great success and she told one of her guests that she had enjoyed every minute of it which shows that she is in good health for one of her age. We had a family luncheon party in her own home—which included four generations. People and flowers poured in and out of the house all day. She had a visit from the B.B.C., the result of which were several broadcasts in which her memories of the Pikes Peak Expedition were recorded. A few weeks ago representatives of the Canadian B.C. visited her in connection with the work she did with Sir William Osler. We contacted her friend, Dr. Cunningham, who called on her birthday accompanied by Professor Whitting. Sir Richard Doll, Regius Professor of Medicine in Oxford University also called. She received over 100 telegrams and cards from all parts of the world, including, of course, that from Her Majesty The Queen.

The local *Oxford Mail* photographed and interviewed her. Some of the most interesting things in her long life were her work on respiration in Colorado and her study with Haldane of alveolar gases in children. She also spoke of the encouragement she got from Osler.

All this roused the University of Oxford. Her neighbor Roger Elliott, who had helped her a lot in the previous fifteen years, worked together with the Regius Professor of Medicine, Sir Richard Doll, to have the university offer her an Honorary Master of Arts degree. Her example, Sir Richard wrote, first convinced Oxford "that women can do as well as men." She received the M.A. at a special congregation held near Christmas 1972 in the Old Congregation House. She was admitted by the vice chancellor, the historian Alan Bullock. Her degree, he acknowledged, came some three-quarters of a century late. With this she made the *London Times* and was famous nationally as the first centenarian to be given an Oxford Master of Arts degree (fig. 3.6).

The *Oxford Mail* of December 14, 1972, reported: "Miss FitzGerald . . . studied physiology at the turn of the century . . . and passed the examinations brilliantly. . . . The public orator Mr. Colin Hardie said in his Latin speech that it was Oxford's fault she had no degree. Miss Fitz-Gerald did so splendidly in an examination that Prof. Gotch at once declared the Honours School of Physiology must be opened to women, and eventually all other schools were opened to them. I have presented one nonagenarian, but I doubt if any centenarian has ever been presented before."

On December 15, the *New York Times* also carried her picture and the story of a woman who was "tough-minded" enough to "return a note from Queen Victoria after marking up the imperfections in phrasing" and who despite "brilliant" work had been denied a degree on the grounds that the university did not then admit women. In response to a reporter's question of her most important work, she simply pointed to a letter from Sir Richard Doll that stated that two out of three medical scholarships recently awarded went to women.

At the request of Bruce Dill (1973), chairman of the Committee for Senior Physiologists of the American Physiological Society, her neighbor Mr. Cannon described the events surrounding the award ceremony:

> She was asked whether she would like a small ceremony at her home or go to a full ceremony. . . . Her prompt answer was, I prefer to go to a full ceremony. We were able to arrange a special ceremony for Miss FitzGerald alone, in the Convocation House adjoining the Sheldonian Theatre. . . . She at once began preparing her list of persons to be invited and her niece and I sent out 180 invitations to persons she knew from all walks of life including Professors, Doctors, Lord Mayor, Chief of Police, etc. It was a really delightful ceremony and approximately 200 persons were present. On entering the Hall, dressed in her cap and gown, she waved to all her visitors on both sides of the Hall and was in very good form. She had many telegrams and letters of congratulations (about 200). To my surprise she asked me to arrange for her to be driven round the city on the journey back to her home as she wished to see any alterations that had been made.

The Physiological Society was aroused by all the publicity, and near Easter 1973 its committee elected her as an ordinary member. She was formally admitted to the society at its annual general meeting on March 24, 1973. Admitted as honorary members at the same meeting were the Nobel laureate Sir Hans Krebs and the famous Italian physiologist Rudolph Margaria. The admission of Mabel FitzGerald was much delayed. She had been ignored when women were first admitted to membership in the United Kingdom Physiological Society during the First World War. She had been a member of the American Physiological Society for sixty years and in 1973 was their oldest living member.

She accepted as a matter of course her Oxford degree and her membership in the Physiological Society—she had worked for them. In the summer of 1973 the university's Final Honour School Examinations in Physiological Sciences—examinations she herself had not been allowed to take for credit—were held and the candidates were asked to comment on a remark in her paper: "The symptoms of oxygen deficiency at high altitudes are therefore due to deficiency, not in the *amount*, but in the *partial pressure* of oxygen in the arterial blood."

She found this quotation and recognition to be a vindication of the quality of her work. She was enormously pleased. The examiners, all of them, had hoped to call on her, but she had become bedridden and she died in her home in August 1973, aged 101.

Number 12 Crick Road contained many interesting FitzGerald papers, and they are now kept in the Bodleian Library, Oxford. FitzGerald herself had worked through many of these, and some have comments on them in her own handwriting. The family had not thrown away any letters and there were boxes of them, a lot from Mabel in New York to her sisters in Oxford; some of these have been quoted here. A long correspondence from Haldane is particularly useful for filling out the details of the Pikes Peak expedition. Together the letters and the scientific papers make a good account of the expedition. FitzGerald probably wanted her story written up someday. Now it has been done, perhaps just in time for catching details that might otherwise be lost. It is a fascinating story to tell about her as a person, and not a piece of dutiful hagiography about a dull scientist dedicated only to research.

In that story a key chapter took place in Colorado's high mountains. It was of an intrepid traveler, an Englishwoman who, by herself, went to the raucous towns and mining camps in 1911 and persuaded the state's early citizens to be subjects for her experiments. She was a pioneer in every sense—in her pursuit of knowledge, her successful efforts to obtain grants and employment, her pleasure trips, and her scientific expeditions. For Mabel Purefoy FitzGerald, Pikes Peak was an adventure, literally the high point in her long life. For those who follow, her legacy is not only an enduring chapter in altitude research, but also the pioneering life of an independent woman who was ahead of her time and thus helped open the doors of scientific education, medicine, and research to women.

Postscript

Torrance's research into FitzGerald's life and career was something of a personal pilgrimage for himself, as his letters to JTR show:

December 19, 1989: "My problem with being the one who knows a lot about Mabel is that I cannot see her as anything but Haldane's research assistant. . . . I see her much more as the last page of an account of the Peak expedition itself."

October 22, 1993: "I was unhappy about publishing my piece on her 20 years ago when I first read up about her [for] a talk to a medical dining club in Oxford. . . . I believed that [she] would hardly appeal to a coldly scientific clinical scientist of 1975. . . . But I think the picture is changing. The history of women in science is being more noticed and she really has got observations to her name."

And now, in the current chapter, Torrance writes: "It is a fascinating story to tell about her as a person, and not a piece of dutiful hagiography about a dull scientist dedicated only to research."

Mabel Purefoy FitzGerald would be pleased at this evolution in her biographer.

Notes

1. This chapter draws heavily on "Mabel's Normalcy," a previous publication by R. W. Torrance (1999). In December of 1998, shortly before his final illness, Robert William Torrance (1923–1999) was pleased to approve a near-final version of this manuscript on Mabel Purefoy FitzGerald. It was the culmination of more than a quarter century of his research into her life and work, and more than a decade of collaboration with me (JTR) for this book. From 1952 until he retired in 1990, Torrance was a fellow of St. John's College, Oxford. His photograph, shown at the beginning of the chapter, was taken in 1994. He died in Oxford on January 8, 1999. His obituary by Charles Michel appeared in Oxford's *Independent*, January 23, 1999.

2. Gerald B. Webb (1871–1948), an English physician, who had come to Colorado Springs to cure his wife of tuberculosis, remained there after her death and devoted the rest of his life to the study of the disease. His counts of the white blood cells in the men on Pikes Peak are given in an appendix to the report (Douglas et al. 1913).

3. Official Colorado highway elevations that differ from some of those reported by FitzGerald are: Denver, 5,280 ft. (1,609 m); Colorado Springs, 6,012 ft. (1,833 m); Ouray, 7,706 ft. (2,349 m); Ridgeway, 6,985 ft. (2,129 m); Telluride, 8,745 ft. (2,665 m); Marshall Pass 10,846 ft. (3,306 m); Mt. Sneffels (FitzGerald wrote "Mount Sueffels"), 14,150 ft. (4,283 m); Uncompahgre Peak (she wrote "Mount Uncompahgré"), 14,309 ft. (4,361 m).

4. Thomas H. Huxley (1835–1895), a friend of Charles Darwin, was an extremely influential biologist and a powerful defender of Darwin's theories of evolution. FitzGerald had her own copy, inscribed with her name and the date of October 1896, of his classical text *Lessons in Elementary Physiology*.

5. Sir William Osler (1849–1919), a Canadian by birth and a classical scholar, was successively professor of medicine at McGill University (1874–1884), University of Pennsylvania (1884–1889), Johns Hopkins University 1889–1904), and Oxford University (1904–1919). He was a consummate clinician and educator, and in 1892 he published his classic, forward-looking textbook, *The Principles and Practice of Medicine*. In the United States he has been considered the "father of modern American medicine." Medical history was one of his great interests, and FitzGerald assisted him in this by collecting old and rare medical books.

6. Hideyo Noguchi (1876–1928) was the brilliant Japanese-born bacteriologist known for his work on syphilis, Oroya fever, and other infections. His work was noticed by Flexner, and in 1904 he joined the Rockefeller Institute in New York City.

7. Simon Flexner (1863–1946) was the famed bacteriologist who under the direction of John D. Rockefeller Sr. and Jr. formed in New York City in 1903 the Rockefeller Institute, which he headed until his retirement in 1935.

8. Archibald B. Macallum (1858–1934) was a distinguished professor of biochemistry at the University of Toronto and founder of the National Research Council of Canada. He, like FitzGerald, was of Scottish heritage.

9. Harvey W. Cushing (1869–1939) was an American neurosurgeon and the first person to operate successfully on the human brain. Part of his training was under Osler at Johns Hopkins, where he was later a faculty member. In 1925 he won the Pulitzer Prize in biography for his book *The Life of Sir William Osler*.

4
AN AFFAIR OF THE HEART
The Grollmans and Cardiac Output on Pikes Peak
Arthur P. Grollman, M.D., and John T. Reeves, M.D.

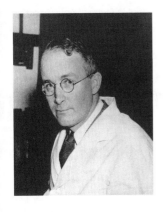

What medical quest would lead a young man to take his bride of three years for much of the summer to the very summit of Pikes Peak? Years later, when his work was severely criticized, had it all gone for naught? Arthur P. Grollman, *left*, and John T. Reeves tell the story of Grollman's parents in this high adventure. As did his father, Grollman got his M.D. degree from Johns Hopkins University and his clinical training in the Johns Hopkins hospital. Since 1974 he has been professor and departmental chairman of pharmacology at the State University of New York at Stony Brook. His field of study has not been the circulation but rather the structure of DNA and how this essential molecule may come to be damaged in disease.

—THE EDITORS

When we go to high altitude, does our heart change the amount of blood it pumps? We feel our hearts race and intuitively we feel a lack of oxygen has stressed our circulation. But has it really happened? Until the summer of 1929 essential details of how the circulation responded to altitude stress were unknown. On Pikes Peak in 1911, J. S. Haldane and his colleagues (chap. 2) had shown a small increase in heart rate and had suggested that the heart's pumping action was not much changed, but their methods were very approximate. It was an important question. For what counts is how much blood the heart pumps each minute—in medical terms, the cardiac output. If the cardiac output is

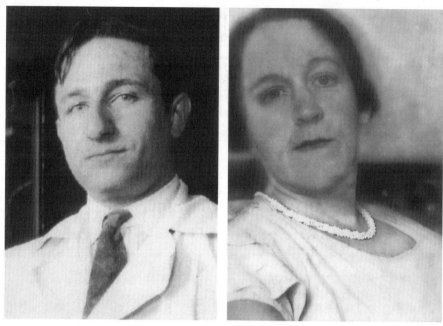

Fig. 4.1. Arthur Grollman and Anna Louise Costello Grollman, 1929. Courtesy
National Library of Medicine and Arthur P. Grollman.

inadequate, increases in breathing and heart rate are useless because
needed oxygen does not reach the tissues. In the summer of 1929 a
husband-and-wife team, Arthur and Anna Louise Grollman (fig. 4.1),
set out for Colorado to work first on the summit and then at the base of
Pikes Peak to learn how much blood the heart pumps at high altitude.
    Intuition could not predict the answer. On one hand, low oxygen
(hypoxia) at altitude could impair the heart's ability to function, maybe
even causing it to fail. Only a few years before, in 1915, this had been
the initial idea of Glover and Newsom (chap. 1). When heart failure
occurred in cattle at high altitude, they thought it was because hypoxia
interfered with the pumping action of the heart muscle. And if heart
muscle contracted poorly at altitude, one would expect the cardiac output would fall. On the other hand, just the opposite might happen. If the
heart muscle worked well at altitude, but if the body was starved for
oxygen, then the heart might pump more blood than normal to compensate for the oxygen lack. Surprisingly, neither scenario proved quite
correct, for nature's picture is often complicated. In one remarkable
summer the Grollmans did what no one had done before—they described
the puzzling changes in cardiac output at altitude. Their findings have

stood the test of time; they have piqued the imagination of subsequent researchers; they have laid a foundation for understanding the heart's response to hypoxia; and, yes, they have yet to be fully explained. So we wonder why this husband-and-wife team sought the pieces of this puzzle, and why they sought them on the summit of Pikes Peak.

With the dawning of new knowledge at the outset of the twentieth century, there were good reasons to examine cardiac output at high altitude, where the oxygen supply was limited. In 1912 a physician, J. B. Herrick, showed for the first time that occlusions of coronary arteries caused heart attacks. Shutting off blood flow and oxygen supply to a portion of the heart muscle could be fatal. Arthur Grollman wondered how the heart would function with less drastic reductions in oxygen supply, a question he felt was important to clinical medicine. In addition, other developments were stimulating worldwide interest in the effects on the body of low-oxygen environments. On December 17, 1903, the Wright brothers had flown the first airplane, and people began to explore the sky in motor-powered aircraft where the pilots and passengers were exposed to the rarified atmosphere. In May 1927, just two years before the Grollmans went to Pikes Peak, Lindbergh had made his famous solo flight across the Atlantic in an unpressurized airplane. In addition mountaineers were beginning to challenge the world's highest peaks, including the assaults on Mt. Everest in 1922 and 1924. Skiers and hikers were probing the mountains, and growing populations of miners and ranchers were living at high altitudes around the world. How did flying, climbing, and living at high altitude affect the pumping action of the heart? The answers were simply not known.

Because the heart is so essential in maintaining oxygen supply to the tissues, two of the world's best physiologists, Haldane on Pikes Peak in 1911 (chap. 2) and Barcroft in Peru in the years 1921–1922, had investigated the cardiac output at high altitude, but the methods were not very precise and their results disagreed. Using his new, simple, and reliable method, Grollman felt he could convincingly answer the questions that had been raised. Further, since he had measured cardiac output in himself and in Anna Louise dozens of times in Baltimore, he already had two experienced subjects and knew exactly their cardiac output values near sea level. And if they could spend their summer vacation in 1928 at Woods Hole on Cape Cod where Arthur sailed on the trawler *Princeton*, making rather esoteric measurements in urine from the (aglomerular) goosefish (Grollman 1929a), why not better spend the summer of 1929 on the summit and at the base of Pikes Peak, measuring cardiac output in themselves?

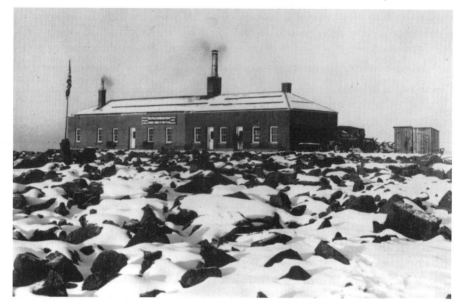

Fig. 4.2. Summit house on Pikes Peak, 1920. Courtesy Colorado Springs Pioneers Museum.

To study how low oxygen affected the heart, Pikes Peak was the ideal laboratory, and Grollman chose it for the same reasons as had Haldane (chap. 2). First of all, there was access from Manitou Springs by automobile and cog railway. Although the summit house that Haldane and his associates had used had burned and a new one had been constructed (fig. 4.2), some repair of the old house may have occurred. According to the article in the *Colorado Springs Gazette and Telegraph* of Sunday, June 30, 1929, the Grollmans "have quarters in the old highway summit house where he has set up a laboratory. . . . Each day he makes about a dozen measurements, some during exercise, . . . some before eating, etc. But most are made early in the morning . . . without disturbance of any kind." If one is to know the effect of high altitude on the heart, then other influences must be avoided, because heart rate and cardiac output are extremely labile. Everyone who has blushed or known the rising tide of anger, shivered in the cold, felt faint on standing up, or counted the pulse after eating or exerting knows that the circulation responds quickly to emotion, temperature, posture, activity, and intake of food or drink. If the effect of altitude itself was to be seen, all of these other factors must be carefully controlled. No one knew this principle better than Grollman. With trainloads of tourists arriving at the top every two hours or so, having a quiet laboratory apart from the hubbub was essential for his purposes. With these Pikes Peak facilities, Grollman could minimize the disturbing extraneous influences. Even the weather cooperated for most of their month on the summit. "Fortunately, Pikes Peak during the first three weeks of the present study was favored with an unprecedented warm and equable climate, . . . and, in general, the climate was comparable to conditions in Baltimore during the late autumn" (Grollman 1930a).

Although the Grollmans lived and worked in a separate building, the amenities of the summit house should not be underestimated. It offered food, warmth, and, not least of all, company. Despite the panorama and glorious sunsets, without conversation with others a self-imposed exile of several weeks on the top of a rocky, barren mountain could be lonely, even for a recently married couple. According to the *Gazette* report, Grollman himself was fully occupied by the experiments. "It takes him so long to analyze the measurements . . . that it requires steady application of the work each day to complete it by dark. . . . Then he has to work throughout the evening to complete the calculations." Although Anna Louise was a constant reader and an inveterate correspondent, Grollman noted that she "endured the long sojourn on the mountain to act as a subject." For social interaction she must have enjoyed talking both to the employees at the summit house and to the steady stream of tourists visiting the Peak. And the conversations were not entirely social, for some of the young, healthy men who were employed at the summit house and some who came as tourists were recruited as subjects. Whereas study of the tourists would show the acute affects of altitude, the employees would show the effects following acclimatization. Because from the subject's point of view Grollman's measurements were simple and not invasive, the more curious and adventurous young men could easily be persuaded to volunteer.

Unlike Haldane's Anglo-American expedition of 1911 to Pikes Peak, which was supported by grants both from the Royal Society in England and from Yale University, Grollman had no grant, and the limited Hopkins Special Research Fund had to be shared among the faculty. In 1929 the National Institutes of Health giving billions annually for medical research did not exist. As an associate in physiology at Johns Hopkins,[1] Grollman's salary was $2,500 a year, so supporting Pikes Peak research from the family budget, as it was necessary to do, was not easy. Furthermore, he was a medical student. Economy was essential, and even much of his equipment was homemade apparatus (fig. 4.3).

On June 20, after going by train to Colorado Springs and traveling for two hours by automobile to the summit of Pikes Peak, Arthur and Anna Louise spent the evening "unpacking and setting up the apparatus."

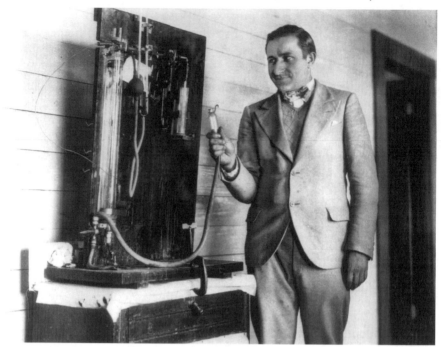

Fig. 4.3. Arthur Grollman with the gas analysis apparatus used for measuring cardiac output. Courtesy of Arthur P. Grollman.

Early the next morning on June 21 they made the first of twenty daily measurements. After the initial three weeks of study on themselves, the weather deteriorated, and during their final week on the summit, marked by "daily electrical storms," they made measurements on tourists and the summit house employees. On about July 22 they descended to Manitou Springs to an altitude of 6,562 feet. While there, even though they measured cardiac output in themselves for another seventeen consecutive days, the pace of the experimental work must have been slower than on the summit, allowing some time for a well-deserved vacation. If Anna Louise had found the summit of Pikes Peak confining, she certainly would have enjoyed idyllic days in Manitou Springs.

By timing their visit to Colorado between the middle of June and the end of August in 1929, the Grollmans may have picked the last window of opportunity for their venture. The storm clouds of national economic disaster were forming, and funding in a subsequent year might have been even more scarce. In July and August of 1929, wealthy Americans and international tourists flocked to Manitou Springs, a premier resort at the pinnacle of its popularity. Fortunately everyone was blithely

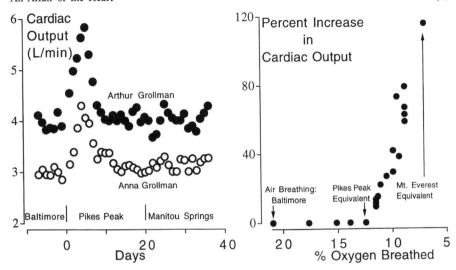

Fig. 4.4. Measurements of cardiac output. Left, the cardiac output values at sea level, on the summit of Pikes Peak (14,110 feet), and after descending to Manitou Springs (6,412 feet) in Arthur Grollman and Anna Louise Grollman. Right, percent increase (compared to breathing sea-level ambient air, 20.93 percent oxygen) in Arthur Grollman's cardiac output when he breathed low-oxygen mixtures for eight to sixty minutes in Baltimore. Reducing oxygen concentration in the air breathed simulates going to altitude, and some representative locations and altitudes are shown. Drawn from data in Grollman 1930a.

unaware that two months later, on October 29, stocks on Wall Street would plummet, presaging the Great Depression. For at least the next decade, money, especially for medical research, would be hard to find. Manitou Springs would never be the same again.

But for Grollman the timing was right. Although he easily recruited subjects on Pikes Peak, the basic design of the experiments called for only two subjects, himself and Anna Louise. Careful, frequently repeated measurements in one or two subjects are far superior to casual, occasional, random, or merely approximate measurements in many subjects, a research principle well known to Grollman. In fact, over a two-year period in Baltimore he made 114 cardiac output measurements in himself (1930b). As a result of these and the many cardiac output measurements in Anna Louise, he knew precisely the normal sea-level values for both of them. As we shall see, he would later be criticized for attempting to apply such strict criteria to others. But, for Pikes Peak, having made these prior measurements was a great advantage because he could compare the values on the summit with those well known from Baltimore.

On Pikes Peak, the daily cardiac output measurements, made the morning after arrival and for the next three weeks, have provided our clearest picture of the changes at altitude (fig. 4.4). It was fortunate he made such daily observations, for the time course of the changes was complex. Compared to sea level, the cardiac output was nearly normal the morning after arrival on the Peak; it rose steadily over the next four to five days and then subsided to sea-level values. Such a complete description could only have been discovered by Grollman's type of experimental design. Although subsequent researchers have made many measurements of cardiac output at high altitude, Grollman's daily time course of changes has yet to be improved, or even duplicated.

Because these findings on the Peak were unexpected, how were they to be interpreted? By invoking teleology, the wisdom of the body, Grollman felt he could understand a "purpose" for a high cardiac output on Pikes Peak. If the heart pumps blood in order to supply the cells of the body with oxygen, then when the oxygen supply becomes limited at high altitude and the blood contains less oxygen, the heart should pump more blood to compensate. At least this would seem a sensible thing for the heart to do.

Using the same reasoning, Grollman also felt he could understand why the increase in cardiac output might be temporary. After day five on Pikes Peak, as he knew from Haldane's 1911 expedition to Pikes Peak and his own results, the body was making other adjustments to the altitude, namely, increases in breathing and in the concentration of hemoglobin in the blood. Both of these adjustments would increase the amount of oxygen in the blood and would reduce the need for the heart to continue to pump so much. In his words, "increased oxygen capacity of the blood [replaces] the increased cardiac output as a means of supplying the tissues with their normal oxygen" (Grollman 1930a).

But why did cardiac output take several days to reach its maximal value on Pikes Peak? He had not expected this and it puzzled him. If the main job of the heart is to pump blood to supply oxygen to the tissues, it should pump more blood on arrival when the blood oxygen is at its lowest level. Yet the cardiac output did not reach its maximal value until several days later, when the blood oxygen level had improved. Grollman had to be content with merely stating the facts: "Low oxygen [in] the inspired air, as encountered at the elevation of Pikes Peak is not in itself an immediate stimulus to an increased cardiac output." Although he had correctly stated the facts, they bothered him.

Maybe he had made an experimental error, but he could find none. Even though Anna Louise had been confined to bed with altitude sickness (headache, loss of appetite, and malaise) for her first two days on the mountain, her changes in cardiac output (fig. 4.4) were the same as in himself. Both before and after Pikes Peak, the control measurements in Baltimore were rock solid for both of them, so there was no problem with the baseline measurements. Tourists who were examined on their fourth or fifth day on Pikes Peak had cardiac output values higher than predicted, but those examined the day of arrival or after a prolonged stay did not. The altitude-acclimatized employees at the summit house did not have elevated cardiac outputs. Everything was consistent; the measurements all pointed to a cardiac output that *"gradually increased during the days following arrival from a low altitude but declines again and resumes its normal sea-level value within about two weeks"* (Grollman's italics). His use of italics emphasized the important and puzzling gradual increase in output after arrival on the Peak.

After he returned to Baltimore from Pikes Peak, the finding continued to bother him. Because cardiac output was not changed from sea level to arrival on Pikes Peak, he reasoned, then the output should not change in Baltimore if for a few minutes he breathed hypoxic air to simulate the ambient air on Pikes Peak. On September 10, within two weeks of his return to Baltimore, he began experiments to see if the acute breathing of simulated "Pikes Peak air" would raise his cardiac output. It did not (fig. 4.4).

But would the heart respond at all when a sea-level resident breathed low-oxygen mixtures for a few minutes? And if so, how low would the oxygen in the air have to go before the pumping action of the heart would increase? On September 11 he performed a dangerous experiment on himself. For eight long minutes he breathed a homemade mixture of air and nitrogen that he felt contained 7 percent oxygen, the equivalent of breathing air at the summit of Mt. Everest. For a sea-level resident unacclimatized to high altitude, breathing air containing so little oxygen causes unconsciousness within seconds and death shortly thereafter. From Haldane's work, he must have known of the insidious nature of severe hypoxia, where the subject may die without even knowing of the danger. Although there may have been slightly more oxygen in the mixture than he thought, still his color became extremely blue, and he reported "loss of mental capacities." With his confusion, had he been unattended, he could have been harmed and he would have been incapable of performing the experiment, so there had to be another person present. For this extreme circumstance, where measurements were somehow obtained, they showed a large increase in cardiac output (fig. 4.4). The heart promptly and vigorously increased its pumping action in response to this sudden crisis of near-total oxygen deprivation.

Another experiment, on November 7, was also courageous, for he breathed a mixture containing less than 9 percent oxygen, equivalent to 22,000 feet, for an entire hour. A less hardy person would have been confused and incapacitated. Today's committees concerned with human research would very carefully prescribe safeguards for subjects breathing such low-oxygen mixtures, but no such advice was available to Grollman. He must have considered some safeguards, for he emerged unscathed from his drastic experiments. With these experiments and others that were less heroic, he demonstrated how the cardiac output would respond acutely over the entire range of oxygen values possible in life for humans (fig. 4.4). The cardiac output did not increase until he breathed low-oxygen mixtures equivalent to 15,000 feet or higher, findings that have since been confirmed (Torre-Bueno et al. 1985; Wagner et al. 1986). In essence, as the oxygen level in the air falls, the heart is capable of acutely increasing its pumping action, but it does not do so until the degree of hypoxia becomes more severe than occurs on Pikes Peak.

In retrospect, as we review Grollman's findings, clearly the ability of the heart to pump blood was not impaired by very low oxygen levels; in fact, it was just the opposite. During the first few days on Pikes Peak cardiac output was increased, not depressed. In contrast to the speculation from 1915 in cattle at 10,000 feet (chap. 1), the heart had not failed at high altitude. With the advent in recent years of heart catheterization and echocardiography, researchers have shown how the heart muscle maintains its ability to contract strongly at high altitude, even up to the summit of Mt. Everest! During severe, acute hypoxia in Baltimore, Grollman's heart pumped vigorously even though he suffered "loss of mental capacities." In the face of severely reduced oxygen levels, the heart is robust, and more so than the brain, a concept that Grollman demonstrated for the first time.

With the measurements on himself on November 7, 1929 (1930a), Grollman concluded his studies on oxygen lack and never again returned to them. On November 12, the editor of the prestigious *American Journal of Physiology* received his paper for publication. Grollman had performed the final measurements, composed the last table of results, drawn a new figure for the manuscript, finished the writing, and mailed it to the editor, who received it in just five days! Not only did Grollman not spare himself, but his capacity for work was clearly prodigious. The paper appeared in 1930. Grollman had concluded "*that there are two essentially different conditions which bring about a cardiac response to anoxemia* [low oxygen in the blood]. There is an *immediate* reaction which shows itself in the course of a few minutes, and a *delayed* reaction (such as was observed on Pikes Peak) which requires many hours for development" (Grollman's italics). Something other than oxygen level was controlling the cardiac output during the first five days on Pikes Peak, and with some prescience Grollman speculated the central nervous system was involved. The issue is still not resolved, but changes with altitude within the sympathetic nervous system may be just the place to look.

So what were the practical implications of Grollman's work on Pikes Peak? As reported in his 1929 interview in the *Colorado Springs Gazette*, he wanted to study heart function in the low-oxygen environment of high altitude. The findings, he said, might have implications in heart disease, "one of the most frequent causes of death." He found the heart to be surprisingly resistant to low levels of oxygen. Also, after acclimatization on Pikes Peak, exercise cardiac output was not greater than at sea level (Grollman 1931b). He commented on the implication for air travelers. Only when persons ascend in "aeroplane flights" higher than 15,000 feet would their cardiac output increase. Unlike Lindbergh, we no longer cross the Atlantic in unpressurized airplanes, but rather in cabins pressurized at 6,000 to 8,000 feet. Based on data from the Grollmans, men and women traveling by air can expect normal cardiac output values during their journey. Although healthy climbers ascending the highest peaks face many grave dangers, heart failure is not one of them because the heart muscle withstands very low oxygen levels and the heart itself is not called upon for an excessive output.

In the body of Grollman's report from Pikes Peak was a statement that has been largely ignored, namely, "unacclimatized persons often show marked . . . nausea or *fainting* after a heavy meal" (italics mine). Possibly a heavy meal in a warm environment combined with altitude was responsible. Having found in Baltimore that a heavy meal caused the heart to markedly increase its pumping action, he probably observed with great interest the occasional fainting in tourists after they had arrived above 14,000 feet via the cog railway and then proceeded to eat heartily in the warm and comfortable summit house restaurant. Researchers in Colorado have recently reported that visitors who have just arrived in Keystone (altitude 9,250 feet) may faint when they stand up after eating a large meal (Nicholas et al. 1992). These investigations have supported Grollman's original findings of what physicians now call "high-altitude fainting." Although the cause is still not known, the phenomenon was well known to Grollman in 1929 on Pikes Peak and was first described by him.

Arthur and Anna Louise Grollman met while taking summer courses at the University of Chicago and married in 1926. He had come from

Baltimore and she from Indianapolis, where she had been born and raised. Although she must have known her intended husband was an intense and ambitious young man, how could Anna Louise have imagined when she met Arthur, a chemist just beginning physiological research, that she would become a subject for his research? She was to be a schoolteacher, not a physiologist. Yet there was already ample evidence of his remarkable work ethic, combined with considerable talent. He had been born in 1901 into an immigrant family of modest means and had worked his way through both high school and college. In 1920, before the age of nineteen, he had received his B.A. degree, Phi Beta Kappa, from Johns Hopkins. In June 1923 he had received his Ph.D. degree in physical chemistry, also from Johns Hopkins. Anna would have known Arthur was an achiever and their life together would bring surprises, but she certainly could not have imagined spending their third summer together in measuring their own cardiac output values above 14,000 feet on the summit of Pikes Peak in Colorado.

Drive and perseverance were part of Arthur Grollman's character. On May 5, 1923, one month before he received his Ph.D., he had sent Dean Williams of the Johns Hopkins School of Medicine a handwritten, two-page letter in which he said: "I write to inquire whether it would be possible for me to obtain an assistantship in the Hopkins Medical School which, while paying a sum sufficient only for a bare subsistence, would also permit me, at the same time, to follow the regular course in medicine. . . . It is now my desire to receive an M.D. degree and thus fit myself for research in the medico-chemical sciences" (1923).

These two sentences were prophetic and relevant to the study on Pikes Peak. The first illustrated Grollman's willingness to sacrifice immediate personal comfort for his long-term goals; the second outlined his strategy of combining medicine and chemistry for a career in research, a strategy that guided the remainder of his life. If Dean Williams had inquired into the author of this letter, he would have found that Arthur at age twenty-one was among the youngest Ph.D. students to graduate from Johns Hopkins University. In any event, on May 9 Dean Williams responded to "Mr. A. Grollman" in eight lines that simply acknowledged receipt of the request and said, "I am afraid that nothing of the kind is likely." Such a prompt dismissal indicated an underestimation of young Grollman's ability and tenacity.

Grollman promptly looked for other ways to obtain his medical degree. After his Ph.D. degree was awarded, he obtained an appointment as an instructor in chemistry at Johns Hopkins University. Although he now had a job, he likely was not satisfied working on the physical chemistry of solutions (Grollman and Frazer 1923, 1925; Grollman 1925), or on bile acids (Macht et al. 1924), which were too far away from medicine. Probably in 1923 he read the new physical chemistry text by a Johns Hopkins physiologist, B. S. Neuhausen, and through him met the department's distinguished chairman and kidney specialist, E. K. Marshall Jr. Immediately, Marshall and Grollman seem to have hit it off. Marshall was twelve years older than Grollman and also had a degree in physical chemistry from Johns Hopkins University. Marshall needed a bright, young, energetic chemist for his ongoing research in kidney function, and Grollman needed a stepping-stone to medical school. In 1924, when Marshall recruited him to the medical school faculty as an instructor in physiology, Grollman got his chance to study medicine. While maintaining his appointment at Johns Hopkins, he began his medical courses, mostly at Johns Hopkins, but during the summers he attended the University of Chicago (1924 and 1925) and the University of Michigan (1926). He received his M.D. degree in 1930 from Johns Hopkins School of Medicine.

For Grollman, applying chemistry to real-life problems in Marshall's laboratory was a great adventure, and it confirmed his intent to do "medico-chemical research." With characteristic energy, he soon published three research papers that supported Marshall's fundamental concept. The kidney is more than just a filter; it actively excretes certain substances (Grollman 1926a, b). In 1926 Marshall promoted Grollman to associate, but he demonstrated confidence in Grollman's research skills in an even more dramatic way. He put Grollman to work on a problem that had challenged the best physiologists around the world, namely, the measurement in human beings of the amount of blood the heart pumps each minute, the so-called cardiac output.

The time was ripe and the need was enormous. If one could not measure the heart's essential function, namely, the amount of blood it pumps, how could physiologists understand the normal heart and how could physicians advise patients with diseased hearts? With different laboratories, different methods, and different experimental conditions giving different answers, the entire field of cardiac output measurement was in disarray. By the early 1920s the appearance of new methods had energized the field of blood circulation to near fever pitch. By then the human heart could be visualized with the X-ray and fluoroscope, arterial pressure was easily measured with a blood pressure cuff, and a new instrument, the electrocardiograph, was revolutionizing clinical cardiology. Needles could be inserted directly into arteries to measure pressure and the content of oxygen in arterial blood. Missing from this startling array of discovery was a method to measure the heart's pumping action. Throughout the world the race was on for a reliable method to measure cardiac output in humans, and Marshall set Grollman to the task.

Why did Marshall, who was a kidney expert, have an interest in the heart? Marshall himself answers the question in his autobiographical notes (1952):

> Interest in cardiac output stemmed from the fact that at Cambridge in 1923, I worked with Barcroft [see note 4, chap. 5] on the cardiac output of man. The method was, I think, not much good. Barcroft had during the war applied the principle proposed by Fick in 1870 [see appendix] for determining cardiac output in unanesthetized goats. . . . I asked Barcroft why not do it in dogs and received the reply that it could not be done as the dog was too emotional and unstable. I disagreed with him. On my return to Baltimore, I took up the problem and performed the first successful experiment on an unanesthetized dog in January, 1924. . . . Naturally, this work led to an attempt to improve methods for determining the cardiac output of man. This work was done with my associate Grollman, who later modified our first method and spent several years working on the subject.

Barcroft's method, which was "not much good," involved the use of an inhaled "foreign" gas, so called because it did not naturally occur in the body. By using such a method, Barcroft and Marshall correctly determined that output rose in themselves when they were shivering from the cold (Barcroft and Marshall 1923). When Marshall subsequently measured cardiac output in trained dogs, the method involved pushing a needle directly through the chest wall into the left and right ventricles for blood sampling (Marshall 1926), a method not suitable for humans.

Because the entire cardiac output flows through the lung, measuring lung blood flow measures output. To get at lung blood flow, one measures how rapidly the flowing blood removes a gas from the lung, and breathing a foreign gas is a good approach. But breathing a foreign gas led to questions that, among others, included its safety, its solubility in blood, the ease and accuracy with which it could be measured, and obtaining a uniform mixture throughout the lung. If the gas removed from the lung could be measured before the recirculating blood brought the dissolved gas back to the lung, the method and calculations would be simplified (see appendix). These were issues of physiology and physical chemistry, and Grollman was the natural choice for the job. As might be predicted, with Grollman on board the project went into high gear. In less than two years many answers to the questions had been found and the necessary apparatus built. These important studies, the foundations for Grollman's future work, were submitted on June 6, 1928, and were published in the *American Journal of Physiology* (Grollman and Marshall 1928; Marshall and Grollman 1928; Marshall et al. 1928). Marshall then returned to his studies on the kidney, leaving Grollman to carry on the cardiac output work alone.

The pace of the research did not slacken. After considering the properties of several gases suitable for human inhalation, Grollman settled on acetylene (1929b). Hydrogen and nitrogen had too little solubility in blood and gave rise to large experimental errors. Ethyl iodide, chloroform, ether, nitrous oxide, and ethylene were too soluble and gave variable results in different individuals. Acetylene provided the best compromise because it had an acceptable taste, it was innocuous for human administration, its blood solubility was adequate but not excessive and not so different among individuals, and its analysis in blood was relatively uncomplicated. By the end of 1928 Grollman had not only completed these studies but had also developed the equations necessary for cardiac output measurement.

When satisfied with the method, Grollman examined cardiac output over a wide range of human conditions, including changes in posture (1928), ingestion of food and fluids (1929d), seasonal variation during basal rest in a single individual (1930b), variation during rest in a population of individuals (1929c), effect of forced breathing (1930c), variation with environmental temperature (1930d), effect of sleep (1930e), effect of the menstrual cycle (1931a), and changes with mild exercise (1931b). Between June 28, 1928, and September 8, 1930, Grollman submitted thirteen full-length, single-authored publications on the cardiac output in humans, and most were published in the prestigious *American Journal of Physiology*. He subsequently summarized these and related studies in his classic monograph, *The Cardiac Output of Man in Health and Disease* (1932). It was a tour de force in clinical investigation. Even more remarkable is that Grollman did all this while he was a full-time medical student working toward his M.D. degree and also a faculty member with teaching and administrative responsibilities. One wonders when he slept.

This vast amount of work in so important an area did not go unnoticed by the medical research community. Although recognition came quickly, it did not go directly to Grollman, but rather to Marshall. On November 21, 1929, Marshall presented the coveted Harvey Lecture, which he titled "The Cardiac Output of Man" (1929–1930). Unquestionably, the Harvey Lectures in New York City and the Silliman Lectures at Yale University were the country's most prestigious medical honors at that time. No matter how democratic the selection committee may have been, it could not very well give such a high honor to a junior faculty member, who was still a medical student. As professor and departmental chairman, Marshall was invited to give the prestigious lecture. To his credit, he acknowledged that the presentation was largely based on Grollman's work, and he gave due credit, including Grollman's work on Pikes Peak.

> This past summer, Grollman from my laboratory went on an expedition to Pike's Peak, Colorado (14,110 feet, 4,300 m) for the purpose of studying the heart output under these conditions with the very accurate acetylene method. The results show clearly that the basal cardiac output is increased during the first days of residence on the Peak, but soon returns to normal. The maximum increase found was about 40 percent. Subsequent experiments in the laboratory have shown that the breathing of low oxygen mixtures does not produce an immediate increase in cardiac output until the inspired oxygen is decreased to about 11 percent.

Perhaps by oversight, or maybe as a sign of the times, Marshall did not mention in his lecture the other key participant in the studies on Pikes Peak. She was Anna Louise Costello Grollman. By the summer of 1929, Anna Grollman was an experienced subject for cardiac output measurements. Her initials, gender, age, height, and weight identify her as a subject in studies on the variation of cardiac output with posture, received for publication in June 1928 (Grollman 1928), one entire year before Pikes Peak. She was also a subject in three other studies using acetylene before Pikes Peak (Grollman 1929a, b, c), and in at least three published studies afterward (Grollman 1930c, d, 1931a). One of these was a detailed study of the cardiac output variation during the menstrual cycle (1931a). It is of interest that she was the first woman ever to have her cardiac output measurements published.

Controversy and Resolution

It is the very nature of research for important experimental results to come under the scrutiny and criticism of later investigators. In this case criticism was not directed at Grollman's conclusions from Pikes Peak, but rather at the acetylene method for all of his cardiac output measurements. In 1929, as Grollman's output work was winding down, W. F. Hamilton, a physiologist then in Louisville, Kentucky, was introducing a new method (Kinsman et al. 1929). Instead of having the subject breathe a foreign gas, the method involved an injection into the blood of an indicator, such as a colored dye, and measuring its concentration as it appeared downstream. When the output was measured in humans, the values were higher than those found by Grollman. Then, in the late 1940s, with the advent of human cardiac catheterization, cardiac output could be measured more directly (see appendix). Again Grollman's values were too low.

On reviewing the matter in 1962, Hamilton felt he could identify the reason why Grollman's measurements were too low. When a foreign indicator, either a dye or a gas, is introduced into the blood to measure cardiac output, the measurements are to be completed before the indicator recirculates. Hamilton had found that indicators begin to recirculate in about fifteen seconds, not the twenty-four seconds claimed by Grollman. By waiting longer than fifteen seconds to make the measurements, he said, Grollman had found falsely low values. Although Hamilton criticized the low output values, he acknowledged that Grollman had wrestled with the problem of recirculation. Also, because the values were off by a constant percentage, a constant factor could be used to correct them, and the patterns of change were reliable. Because Hamilton found that the normal human cardiac output varied rather widely among individuals, he complained that Grollman had made the normal range of values too narrow, that is, within "Procrustean limits."

Unquestionably, Grollman, known for the care with which he made measurements, had been tenacious in holding on to the accuracy of his method for cardiac output. Julius Comroe, the director of the Cardiovascular Research Institute in California, felt strongly that Grollman's tenacity had been obstructive of scientific progress. In his 1977 philosophical treatise on medical discovery he cited Grollman by name in a chapter entitled "How to Delay Progress Without Even Trying." The chapter described several scientists who, by being eminent and forceful in an erroneous idea, thereby delayed progress. When cardiac catheterization was introduced and cardiac output could be measured more directly, Comroe stated, Grollman's acetylene method, "found to give values far too low, went to its grave."

Comroe's obituary was both premature and ironic. As we shall see, the prematurity relates to the current popularity of modified acetylene methods for measuring cardiac output in humans, even beyond the earth's atmosphere in orbiting spacecraft. The irony is that Comroe's very own laboratory (then in Philadelphia) in the late 1950s (Cander and Foster 1959) and early 1960s (Johnson et al. 1960) was responsible for much of the rehabilitation in physiology and medicine of the acetylene method for the measurement of cardiac output in man. Because Comroe's help and encouragement were acknowledged in the published papers, he obviously knew about these studies from his own laboratory. Then what did Comroe mean when he said Grollman's method has "gone to its grave," and why did it give values "found to be far too low"?

To get the answers to these questions, we turned to Robert L. Johnson Jr., who for nearly four decades has used acetylene for the measurement of cardiac output. In one of those coincidences that punctuate the history of medical research, Johnson had worked on the acetylene method in Comroe's laboratory in the late 1950s and early 1960s. Subsequently he joined the faculty of the Southwestern Medical School in Dallas where Grollman was professor of experimental medicine. Knowing both Comroe and Grollman well and being an expert in the acetylene method, Johnson can give a balanced view of the controversy. His views (1998) are summarized below. More details are given in the appendix.

> In a well designed set of experiments in 1950, Chapman found, in persons undergoing cardiac catheterization, that cardiac output values by Grollman's acetylene method were underestimateet al. et al. d by 25 to 30%. Although the errors in the Grollman method appeared to be cumulative, they were relatively fixed percentages of the true cardiac output. Thus, results by his method correlated closely with those obtained more directly at catheterization.
>
> Probably as a result of the controversy, Grollman has received insufficient credit for his innovations. His ideas were ingenious—the use of rebreathing to improve mixing of gas within the lung, the introduction of acetylene, the development of the mathematical equations, and a design to measure cardiac output under reproducible basal conditions from which the effects of various interventions, such as the effects of high altitude, could be studied. The modifications in Grollman's original method, which have served to rehabilitate the acetylene method for cardiac output measurement, are presented in the appendix. Currently, we might say from the accumulated experience that what has disappeared ("gone to its grave") from the original descriptions are, principally, the use of rebreathing intervals which are too long and the neglect of lung tissue as a reservoir from which acetylene absorption is occurring during rebreathing. Perhaps it is more appropriate to say that Grollman's acetylene method has not disappeared, but has been improved [see appendix] and validated. (Hsia et al. 1995)

Currently not only is acetylene used to measure cardiac output but it is also used for highly specialized medical tests such as pulmonary tissue volume, lung capillary blood volume, lung diffusing capacity (Johnson et al. 1960), and the distribution of ventilation and blood flow in the lung (Wagner et al. 1987). Measurements that have included acetylene have been made at sea level and at various altitudes (Saltin et al.

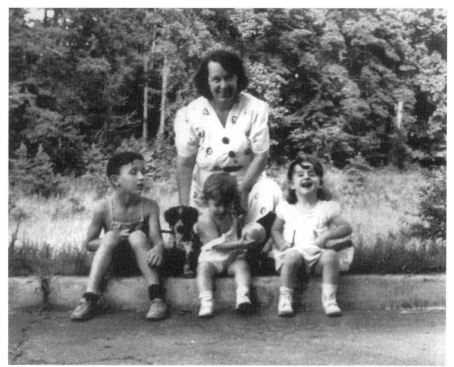

Fig. 4.5. Anna Grollman with her children; from left to right, *Arthur P. Grollman, Catherine Ann Grollman Lauritsen, and Evelyn Frances Grollman, 1940. Courtesy of Arthur P. Grollman.*

1968), including the equivalent of the summit of Mt. Everest (Wagner et al. 1987). Recently acetylene was employed during spaceflight to assist in the measurement of cardiac output as well as pulmonary tissue volume and capillary blood volume (Verbanck et al. 1997). Arguably, acetylene methods are the most reliable of those currently available for the noninvasive measurement of cardiac output at rest and during exercise in normal humans. As modified, the acetylene method has not "gone to its grave," and the measurements on Pikes Peak still stand as the most detailed analysis of the time course of cardiac output changes at altitude. The pioneering studies of Arthur Grollman have left us an important legacy.

Epilogue

Although Arthur and Anna Louise Grollman did not do further work at high altitude, Arthur did a follow-up study in the years 1930–1931. Supported by a Guggenheim Fellowship, Grollman had gone to the Max

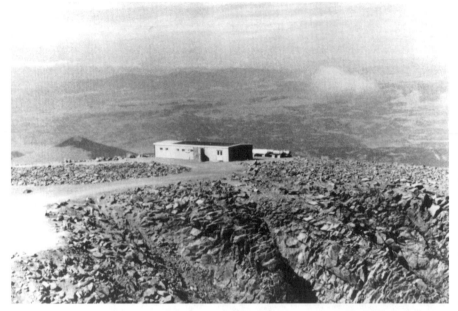

Fig. 4.6. Aerial view of the summit of Pikes Peak, showing the Maher Memorial high-altitude laboratory of the United States Army Research Institute of Environmental Medicine, ca 1965. Courtesy of A. Cymerman, USARIEM, Natick, Massachusetts.

Planck Institute in Heidelberg, Germany, to work with the great German biochemist and Nobel laureate Otto Meyerhof. While in Germany, he initiated a collaborative project with the German physician Baumann, who, for the first time, had measured cardiac output in humans by the direct Fick principle. Baumann's technique required cardiac and arterial punctures. Baumann and Grollman compared the two methods in patients and considered they yielded similar results (Baumann and Grollman 1930).

Many years later the opportunity arose for Grollman to contribute directly to developments in the use of acetylene for cardiac output and high-altitude research, as reported by Robert L. Johnson Jr. (1994) to one of the authors (APG):

> I knew your father [Arthur Grollman] well. He helped me to obtain several grants from the Air Force to study high altitude acclimatization, resulting in two publications involving a modified acetylene technique for measuring pulmonary blood flow [Degraff et al. 1970; Saltin et al. 1968]. It wasn't until later that we began to use a rebreathing technique which we validated against the dye dilution method (Triebwaser 1977). More recently we have validated the

method against the direct Fick (the "gold standard" method for cardiac output in humans) . . . at rest and heavy exercise [Hsia et al. 1995]. The acetylene technique and direct Fick give results that are not significantly different.

Although Grollman did not participate in high-altitude research after Pikes Peak, he was gratified to see the successful modifications of his original acetylene technique, for Johnson and his colleagues used acetylene for cardiac output in health and disease in humans and in animals.

After Pikes Peak the Grollmans remained for several years in Baltimore, where their three children were born (fig. 4.5). In 1932 Marshall left physiology to become chairman of the Department of Pharmacology and Experimental Therapeutics at Johns Hopkins. He brought Grollman along with him into the department. The Grollmans left Baltimore in 1941 and spent most of the war years at Bowman-Gray in North Carolina, where Arthur was research professor of medicine. Thereafter they moved to Texas, where Arthur spent the remainder of his career, chairing in turn the Departments of Physiology and Pharmacology (1946–1950), Biochemistry (1947–1948), and Experimental Medicine (1950–1966).

During his long, active research career, which spanned forty-five years until 1967, he published nearly four hundred papers on a variety of subjects, including the kidney, systemic blood pressure and hypertension, and the endocrine system. Throughout, as in his early days at Hopkins, he retained his interest in the kidney. As a result of his work on high blood pressure he developed a novel treatment for acute kidney failure, namely, the removal of urea and potential toxins by rinsing out the abdominal cavity, a treatment known as intermittent peritoneal lavage. This was a forerunner of the artificial kidney and resulted in his nomination for the Nobel Prize in physiology or medicine and his receipt in 1967 of the Hunter Memorial Award of the American Therapeutic Society. Arthur Grollman died in Dallas on January 31, 1980; Anna Louise lived until 1990.

The Grollmans might be surprised at the magnitude of the scientific legacy left from their summer on Pikes Peak. They would undoubtedly be pleased to have so many of their basic findings from 1929 be substantiated, including the following: (a) The cardiac output rises after one goes from sea level to Pikes Peak; (b) it rises both in men and in women; (c) there is a complex time course to the rise, which indicates it is not simply due to the degree of hypoxemia; (d) the rise is temporary, for with continued stay at altitude the output falls to, or even below, sea-level values; (e) the fall in the output with continued altitude stay is

related in part to the improved oxygen-carrying capacity of the blood
as the subjects acclimatize by increasing breathing and blood hemoglobin concentration; (f) with acute hypoxia the cardiac output does not
rise until the degree of hypoxia becomes severe; (g) the cardiac output
response differs for acute and for chronic hypoxia. Not bad for a month's
stay on Pikes Peak to have so many experimental observations stand
the test of time! The observations the Grollmans made are still important because serial daily measurements have not subsequently been done
in subjects from the day of arrival until acclimatization is complete.
And such measurements are not feasible on major Himalayan expeditions because climbers are well acclimatized on arrival at base camp.

The work of Arthur and Anna Louise Grollman on Pikes Peak opened
a whole field of research with implications for the well-being of people
living at all altitudes. The United States Army, understanding the importance of the heart and circulation at high altitude, has built a permanent laboratory for human research on the summit of Pikes Peak
(fig. 4.6). In that laboratory each summer young men and women live
on the Peak, participating as subjects in high-altitude medical research.
It is a tradition that goes back to the expeditions of Haldane in 1911,
and to the Grollmans in 1929. Efforts to understand Grollman's question of how much blood the heart pumps at high altitude continue.

Appendix—
Basis for and Modifications to Grollman's Method for Measurement of Cardiac Output

The principle (based on the law of conservation of mass) for measurement of cardiac output per unit time, as proposed in 1870 by Adolph Fick,
stated that the amount of oxygen (O_2) brought to the lungs in the venous
blood (the cardiac output times the venous O_2 content) plus the O_2 added
to the blood in the lungs (the O_2 uptake) must equal the O_2 leaving the
lungs in the arterial blood (cardiac output times arterial O_2 content).
Although this "direct Fick" method is considered the "gold standard" for
cardiac output in humans, it is invasive, because sampling the mixed
venous blood requires catheterization of the pulmonary artery, and
sampling the arterial blood requires arterial puncture.

The Fick principle can also be used to measure cardiac output following the inhalation of foreign gases. If the measurements can be completed
before the circulation returns any foreign gas to the lungs, then the venous
content of the gas is zero, and there is no need to sample venous blood. If
the foreign gas comes into equilibrium with the capillary blood in the lung
alveoli, then arterial content of the gas can be calculated from gas alveolar partial pressure and solubility, and there is no need to sample arterial
blood. Therefore a foreign gas method may be noninvasive, as Grollman
realized.

Robert L. Johnson has performed a detailed mathematical analysis of the Grollman method and its current modifications (1998). His full analysis may be obtained from him or the authors. Excerpts are given below:

Grollman's ingenious method substantially improved the foreign gas (nitrous oxide) method as performed by Krogh and Lindhard (1912) which required considerable exertion during complicated respiratory maneuvers. Their method required an accurate breath hold time, measurement of lung volume; and it could not be carried out under reproducible basal conditions. Even in normal subjects the method was subject to errors from uneven distribution in the lung of inspired gas and uneven sampling from different regions of the lung.

Grollman's rebreathing method assured good mixing of the gas within the lungs and between the bag and the lung. Under basal conditions, O_2 uptake was measured by the usual collection of expired air, followed immediately by switching to a bag containing an acetylene gas mixture, which the subject rebreathed. During rebreathing, gas was sampled at the mouth at end expiration after about fourteen seconds and again after about twenty-four seconds. Fractional alveolar O_2 concentration and fractional acetylene concentration were measured in the two gas samples to calculate the changes in alveolar O_2 and acetylene between fourteen and twenty-four seconds. Grollman used these measurements to estimate the arterial to venous O_2 difference across the lungs as calculated from simultaneous changes in O_2 and acetylene concentrations during rebreathing. Using this method of calculation, no measurement was required of the duration of rebreathing or of lung volume. The arterial to venous O_2 difference was referred back to the O_2 uptake measured under basal conditions just prior to rebreathing in order to calculate basal cardiac output.

In 1959 Cander and Forster reported that Grollman had not taken account of acetylene absorption by lung tissue. They pointed out that acetylene rapidly dissolves in the fine septal tissues of the lung which acts as a reservoir into which acetylene disappears in addition to the bag and air dead space volumes; hence, the reservoir from which acetylene is disappearing is the volume of lung-bag system plus the lung tissues. If the tissue volume (which in adults is 500 to 1000 ml) is ignored, the volume of acetylene that has disappeared into the blood will be underestimated by as much as 10 percent, causing a similar underestimate of cardiac output.

Therefore, a major modification of Grollman's technique is the inclusion of an insoluble reference gas which will facilitate the measurement of tissue volume and it is this tissue volume term which has modified Grollman's original equation. The other modifications involve shorter rebreathing times of ten to fifteen seconds at rest and eight to ten seconds during exercise, and the use of rapid gas analyzers to measure breath by breath changes in acetylene concentration [DeGraff et al. 1970; Triebwaser et al. 1977; Barazanji et al. 1996]. With these modifications of Grollman's acetylene method, cardiac output measurements are as reliable as those obtained at cardiac catheterization using the "gold standard" Fick method.

Note

1. An associate in physiology is probably equivalent to the academic rank of assistant professor today, although the *Colorado Springs Gazette and Telegraph* on June 30, 1929, referred to him, possibly in error, as an "associate professor of physiology." According to his own curriculum vitae, Grollman lists his movement up the academic ranks from instructor in chemistry (1923), to instructor in physiology (1924), to associate in physiology (1926), to associate professor of physiology (1931).

5
HIGH CYCLING
Bruce Dill Exercises Harvard Men at the Leadville Fish Hatchery

John T. Reeves, M.D., David Bruce Dill Jr., M.A., and Robert F. Grover, Ph.D., M.D.

Why would a Harvard scientist study men during cycle exercise in the Leadville fish hatchery and how did the experience shape the scientist's future life? David B. Dill Jr. helps tell the story. When young David was growing up, he spent much time in his father's Harvard Fatigue Laboratory and was often an experimental subject for treadmill exercise. For the research project in the summer of 1929, when he was ten, the whole family went to Leadville. He loved the mountains. When he became a geologist, he worked in mines in the United States, Mexico, Canada, Europe, and Chile at altitudes up to 17,000 feet.

—THE EDITORS

"Hello, I'm Bruce. May I join you? I have a suggestion for you young fellows." With this affable greeting, David Bruce Dill, a tall, slender, smiling man in his seventies with cropped white hair (fig. 5.1), introduced himself at breakfast to us, Grover, thirty-eight, and Reeves, thirty-four. It was in June 1963 during a lung conference in Aspen, Colorado, where Dill was one of the speakers. We were surprised and of course flattered to be noticed by one of the world's premier physiologists, and it soon became clear Dill had done his homework. He knew about Grover's research among the high-school students in Leadville, Colorado (chap. 1). Somehow he also knew Reeves was then working at the University of Kentucky in Lexington (altitude 1,000 feet) and had trained with Grover in Denver, so he asked, "Why don't you young fellows collaborate in a study of high-school trackmen, where Lexington athletes would come from low altitude to Leadville for a high-altitude meet, and then the Leadville athletes would go to Lexington for a track meet at low altitude? Not only would there be the element of competition,

111

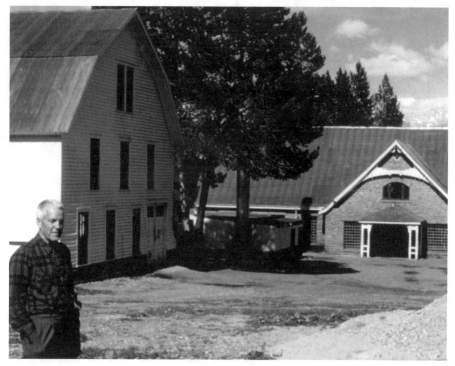

Fig. 5.1. D. Bruce Dill, seventy-three, revisiting the Leadville Fish Hatchery, July 1964. The Hatchery, established in 1889, remains one of the oldest federal hatcheries still in operation in the United States. Dill's 1929 research laboratory was located on the second floor of the white "storage barn" shown behind Dill. Photograph by John T. Reeves.

but also an opportunity to measure performance in the laboratory during altitude acclimatization." With these few words he laid out for us a whole plan of study.

How could we refuse? As the former director of the Harvard Fatigue Laboratory, not only was Dill one of the fathers of exercise physiology, but he was also a pioneer of altitude research in the United States. The project was an opportunity for us to continue our collaboration, which had begun in Denver several years before; it was also novel and sounded like fun. We didn't know it at the time, but this was quintessential Dill, ever eager to stimulate and encourage younger colleagues in research, even people whom he had not previously met, like us. Certainly for us it was the most exciting breakfast at the conference.

Why would Dill want two "young fellows" to do a research project on athletes in Leadville? On looking back at that breakfast meeting, we think the idea began thirty-four years earlier, in 1929, when to an improvised laboratory in the Leadville fish hatchery Dill had brought investigators from Harvard University's Fatigue Laboratory and had examined exercise performance at altitude more closely than anyone had done before (Dill et al. 1931). Although the project had been a great success, was there a loose end, an unanswered question that had been nagging him all these years? We think there was. We believe the question was, "How does acclimatization to altitude affect exercise performance?" To understand why he would ask the question, we must examine why he went to Leadville in 1929 and what he found there.

To put matters in perspective, there was only one laboratory in the United States, and perhaps in the world, dedicated to the scientific study of human exercise in 1929, and that was the Harvard Fatigue Laboratory, with Dill as its head. As implied by the word "fatigue," the laboratory was interested in the limits of human exercise performance. Exercise science was then in its infancy. Only seven years earlier, a Nobel Prize went to the English physiologist A. V. Hill "for his discovery relating to heat production in the muscles."[1] Hill visited Dill and the nascent Harvard Fatigue Laboratory in 1927. Hill had been a runner in his college days and had recently published a basic new principle for human exercise: When oxygen uptake reaches its maximum, the capacity for exercise is at its limit (Hill et al. 1924). The concept that maximal oxygen uptake determines exercise performance was not lost on the Fatigue Laboratory.

Hill also stimulated Dill to think about exercise performance at high altitude. When Hill breathed air diluted with nitrogen, he could take up less oxygen and do less work. But Hill had breathed his air-nitrogen mixture for only a few minutes. What about persons who had been at high altitude long enough to become acclimatized? Perhaps after acclimatization the increase in breathing and blood hemoglobin level would maintain maximal oxygen uptake and exercise capacity at sea-level values. Haldane had studied exercise on Pikes Peak (chap. 2), but he had not measured maximal oxygen uptake or exercise capacity; furthermore an altitude of 14,110 feet might exceed the body's ability to compensate for the reduced amount of oxygen in the air. Dill determined to find out how altitude affected human exercise by leading an expedition, but to a site lower than Pikes Peak.

We can guess why Dill chose Leadville. It was, and still is, a community where people live and work at the moderate altitude of 10,150 feet, and this gave medical relevance to Dill's project. Leadville was more accessible by road and rail than Pikes Peak. In contrast to the Peak, it was well below the tree line, offering a less harsh, more attractive

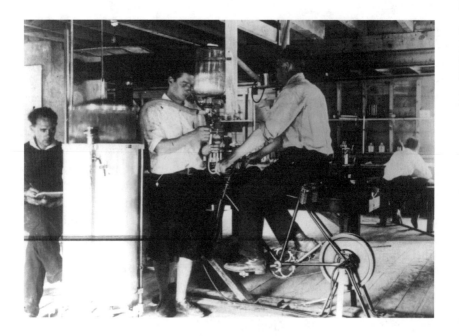

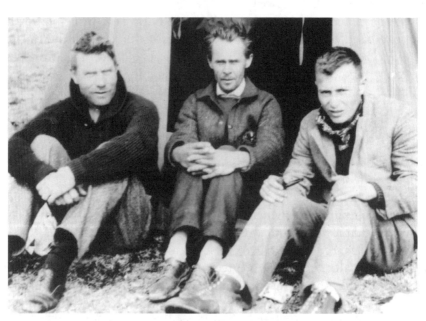

Fig. 5.2. Subjects and the laboratory settings. Top, a subject exercising on the cycle ergometer in the 1929 laboratory on the second floor of the "storage barn." Site identification by Duane Monk, current superintendent of the Leadville Fish Hatchery. Bottom, left to right: Fölling, Oberg, and Pappenheimer, who camped at 14,000 feet on Mt. Elbert during their four-day stay to study the effects of altitude higher than Leadville. Photographs courtesy of D. B. Dill Jr.

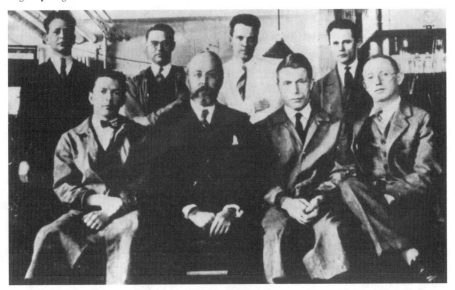

Fig. 5.3. Harvard Fatigue Laboratory staff in 1929. Front row, left to right: John Talbott, L. J. Henderson, A. Fölling, and A. V. Bock. Back row, left to right: W.O.P. Morgan, Harold Edwards, D. B. Dill, and S. A. Oberg. Talbott, Fölling, Edwards, Dill, and Oberg participated in the 1929 Leadville study. Photo from Dill 1967.

environment (fig. 5.1). Finally, the fish hatchery buildings could house the laboratory.

As we shall see, no one at Harvard could be better connected to the United States Fish Commission than Dill, who had been a specialist in fish investigations on the West Coast. Negotiating research space for a summer project at the Leadville hatchery was as simple as talking to an old friend. From the top down, he secured the assistance of the national commissioner and of Mr. Van Atta, the local superintendent in Leadville, and his staff. In 1920 workmen had built a substantial three-story barn with a sawmill on the first floor to provide lumber for subsequent construction (fig. 5.1). Whether the sawmill operated in the summer of 1929 is not known, but the second floor, which was sturdy and spacious, was available. What could have been better? Dill and his colleagues had, free of charge, a heated, 50-by-40-foot laboratory with running water and electric power (fig. 5.2). Although Leadville itself is high, it is actually in the valley of the Arkansas River and is surrounded by mountains more than 14,000 feet tall, including Mt. Elbert, the tallest in Colorado. Some of the team spent four days camped high on Mt. Elbert to make measurements there (fig. 5.2). For reasons of aesthetics, economy, logistics, and science the choice of Leadville was ideal.

L. J. Henderson, the departmental chairman, and A. V. Bock, Dill's mentor, were both strong supporters of the plan.[2] Fielding an enthusiastic research team for Leadville was easy. Of the laboratory's eight members (fig. 5.3), Dill, Fölling, Oberg, Talbott, and Edwards volunteered to go. In addition Dill recruited Alwin M. Pappenheimer, twenty-one, a brilliant recent Harvard graduate (fig. 5.2), who drove his own car to Leadville.[3] As an indication of Dill's inclusive management style, of the eight men from low altitude, all of whom would serve as subjects, six were listed as authors on the published research paper (Dill et al. 1931).[4]

For comparison with the Boston men, Dill recruited three Leadville residents from the hatchery staff. After the eight Boston men had been in Leadville several days, breathing measurements showed them to be as well acclimatized as the three Leadville residents. But measurements that were uncomfortable or invasive, for example, bicycle exercise to maximal effort (fig. 5.2) or arterial puncture during exercise, were done only in the men from the Fatigue Laboratory. Whatever the procedure, Dill was certain to be the first subject.

As Dill commented, the expedition was "principally concerned with muscular activity." After two weeks in Leadville, Dill's own exercise capacity was 20 percent less than it had been in Boston (fig. 5.4A). After six weeks, Talbott's had fallen a similar amount. Edwards's findings were somewhat different, for after four weeks his capacity was nearly 40 percent less than at sea level. Dill must have been surprised, for he tested Edwards repeatedly over the next month, during which interval performance improved, but not quite to the sea-level value. All three men were below their sea-level performance. Even at the moderate Leadville altitude of 10,150 feet, acclimatization had not prevented a fall in their capacity to perform exercise. Dill wrote that exercise "capacity *may* be decreased by one-fifth in normal men at an altitude of 10,000 feet" (italics ours).

Dill's tone was tentative because he wasn't sure. Edwards's exercise capacity had decreased by only 8 percent. What accounted for his steady improvement from the fourth to the eighth week? Talbott also showed a slight improvement from the third to the sixth week. As they continued longer in Leadville, were these men continuing to acclimatize? Dill seems to have thought so, for he commented that the findings in Edwards's case were "apparently associated with acclimatization." Another subject, Oberg, was to have had measurements of maximum oxygen uptake, but a bad knee interfered with his ability to cycle. So, in this instance, Dill was left with only three subjects, and he wasn't sure

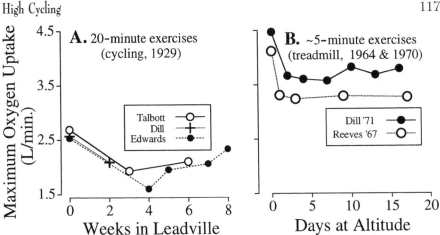

Fig. 5.4. Measurements of maximal oxygen uptake. Panel A (left). In 1929 Dill found maximal values were lower in Leadville than in Boston (time zero). Because no measurements were made immediately on arrival in Leadville, the early time course of the fall was not known. Redrawn from Dill et al., Adaptations of the Organism to Changes in Oxygen Pressure (1931). Panel B (right). The maximal values fell on arrival at high altitude and did not change thereafter, either in Leadville in 1964 or on White Mountain, at 10,100 feet, in 1970. Note that maximal exercises lasting about five minutes give higher oxygen uptake values than do the twenty-minute exercises.

whether exercise performance improved as they acclimatized. He needed exercise measurements immediately on arrival at altitude and then after a long stay, and he didn't have this for a group of subjects.

In 1935 Dill was at altitude again, but it was not possible for him to measure exercise performance during the whole process of altitude acclimatization. In the first place, his participation in the expedition was almost by accident. When Ancel Keys,[5] an enterprising young man who had worked in Copenhagen with August Krogh[6] and in Cambridge, England, with Joseph Barcroft,[7] joined the Harvard Fatigue Laboratory in 1933, he was already planning an international high-altitude expedition. But Keys's negotiations for a high-altitude site in the Himalayan Karakoram collapsed, and the whole project nearly foundered.

Even though I (DBD Jr.) was only ten, I vividly remember Edwards coming to our house on a Saturday afternoon and breaking the news to my father that the Nepalese government had refused a permit for the Fatigue Laboratory to mount an expedition to the Himalayas. Typically

Bruce reacted immediately with ideas for a substitute site, which turned out to be the Chilean Andes. Although he had originally declined to participate, Bruce felt that the reputation of the laboratory was at stake and, reversing his decision, joined the effort. Three members of the Leadville team, Dill, Talbott, and Edwards, participated in what became the famous 1935 expedition to Chile (Dill 1980).

The Chilean expedition was not designed to examine exercise capacity immediately on arrival at high altitude, for the logistics would have been too difficult, but it did reexamine the magnitude of the decrease in men coming from sea level. E. H. Christensen, a talented student of Krogh's, confirmed that maximal oxygen uptake and exercise capacity fell at altitude, and the higher the altitude, the greater was the fall. There was no question that going to altitude interfered with exercise capacity, but the question of whether one performed better after acclimatization than on arrival was still hanging.

However, a way to get at this question may have suggested itself as Dill observed the activities of high-altitude Chilean natives. While working in the mines, young men carried heavy loads uphill with seeming ease. Then, after a full day's work, they played soccer with astounding vigor. After living at altitude for so many years, they surely were well acclimatized. Why not compare exercise capacity in lifelong altitude residents and newcomers?

Having had at the back of his mind for some thirty-four years the question of whether exercise performance at altitude would improve with acclimatization, Dill could easily lay out a study plan to us in 1963 that could provide an answer. We should, he said, simply compare young men living in Leadville with those living at low altitude in Lexington, Kentucky, and make the comparison at both locations. We were willing accomplices. In 1964 we conducted the studies in Leadville and Lexington, and, following his suggestion, we made measurements during maximal exercise on arrival at altitude and serially thereafter. Dill even came to Leadville to see how the project was going (fig. 5.1). While there, he wanted to have his arterial blood sampled during exercise, but the artery in his arm had been hardened into a stone pipe by so many entries over the years, and neither of us could put a needle into it.

On arrival in Leadville in 1964, our subjects decreased their maximal oxygen uptakes by about 20 percent, but there was no improvement during the subsequent seventeen days of acclimatization (Reeves et al. 1967; fig. 5.4B). As for the Leadville athletes, following their descent to low altitude in Lexington, their exercise performance increased just as much as the Lexington athletes' had decreased following ascent to high altitude (Grover et al. 1967). In other words, even with acclimatization to Leadville's altitude from birth, the exercise capacity of these young men was impaired just as much as that of the newcomers from Lexington. In the competition the Lexington men, being superior trackmen, handily won the track meets both in Leadville and in Lexington. Obviously the acclimatized Leadville men did not perform better than those from Lexington, at high or low altitude, on the track or in the laboratory. Altitude dwellers of European descent did not show the athletic prowess Dill had seen in the Andean natives. Dill was both disappointed and unconvinced.

Maybe our men were not sufficiently good athletes, or perhaps we had made a mistake. In any event, in 1970 he repeated much of the study he had suggested to us (Dill and Adams 1971), this time bringing high-school athletes from sea level to White Mountain in California. The altitude of 10,100 feet was similar to that at Leadville, 10,150 feet. There was no native group of altitude residents for comparison with the men from sea level, but otherwise our 1964 study and his of 1970 were practically identical. The findings were also the same—little or no improvement in maximal oxygen uptake as the men acclimatized to altitude (fig. 5.4B). Even so, he didn't give up. In some five studies, in one way or another, he examined exercise performance serially after arrival at altitude, and each time his subjects failed to show the expected improvement. What good was acclimatization if it didn't facilitate exercise at altitude? There was a piece missing from the puzzle.

What was it? Some have suggested Edwards was not well on arrival in Leadville. Because exercise tests were reported for others, but not for him, during his first four weeks there, he could have been recovering. Thereafter, as his health improved, so would his exercise capacity, and this would have accounted for his amazing improvement. But Dill, always careful to mention exceptional circumstances in individuals, made no mention of illness in Edwards.

Even though the results in Edwards remain unexplained, there is at least one other possibility. Dill may have been using an endurance-type exercise in 1929, because his subjects pedaled at the maximum load they could maintain for twenty minutes. Particularly for exercises of long duration, maximum effort depends heavily on subject motivation and is therefore subjective. In his first Leadville trial, Edwards may not have given his best effort. In later years, when we, and Dill himself, used exercises lasting about five minutes, the exercises were much heavier. And assessing maximal effort can be objective (Hill et al. 1924). Furthermore, these shorter exercises give higher maximum oxygen uptakes, as shown by comparison of fig. 5.4A with 5.4B. Using these briefer, heavier exercises, maximum oxygen uptake at altitude does not improve even with months of acclimatization. But endurance has been reported to improve with acclimatization (Fulco et al. 1998), which may in part account for Dill's confusing findings in Edwards in 1929.

Dill's larger question about how and whether altitude acclimatization affects exercise still stands. There are important issues yet to be resolved. How should athletes train for competition at altitude? When they train at altitude for competition at sea level, is this an advantage? Why do football teams from sea level lose much more frequently when they compete in the mile-high city of Denver than at lower altitudes? Does acclimatization facilitate physical or mental work? Are persons with heart disease or hypertension at greater risk if they exercise at high altitude before they are acclimatized? Currently these are questions under intense study. Dill's 1929 study of exercise in Leadville, where people live and work, and his subsequent investigations into the value of acclimatization have opened new fields for scientific inquiry and have laid the foundations for further research.

There was so much more to Dill's 1929 Leadville study that we cannot leave it at this point. Dill fired a final shot, essentially ending the scientific war between Haldane and Barcroft (chap. 2), which was still raging. Haldane believed the lung could actively pump (secrete) oxygen from the air into the blood, but Barcroft didn't accept it. He and the Kroghs believed oxygen molecules simply moved passively across the lung membranes from the air to the blood. Barcroft felt his Peru expedition had disproved Haldane's theory. But Haldane had bitterly complained that Barcroft had miscalculated the reaction between oxygen and hemoglobin in Peru and had falsely rejected the secretion theory (Haldane 1927). In 1929 the war was not only continuing, but it was now being fought on two fronts—whether oxygen was being pumped into the blood and whether altitude altered the reaction of oxygen with hemoglobin.

Dill and his group were able to clarify both issues. Haldane was right about altitude having but little effect on how oxygen binds to hemoglobin. Dill had confirmed it in Leadville and from measurements in Pappenheimer, Fölling, and Oberg during their stay at 14,000 feet on Mt. Elbert (fig. 5.2). But Haldane was wrong about the active "pumping" (secretion) of oxygen from air into blood. Dill found there was "no evidence of secretion of this gas." Not being a combatant in this scientific war, Dill could be impartial. Having overcome Haldane's objection, having accurate methods to analyze the lung air and arterial blood, and studying both rest and exercise in several subjects at low and high altitude, Dill effectively declared Barcroft winner in the war over lung oxygen secretion.

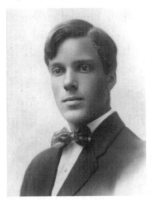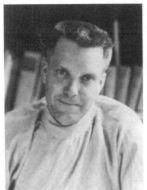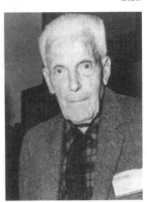

Fig. 5.5. Left to right, *Bruce Dill while a student at Occidental College, California (photograph courtesy of D. B. Dill Jr.); at age forty-eight at the Harvard Fatigue Laboratory (photograph courtesy of Steven M. Horvath); and at age ninety-five during presentation of the Daggs Award (courtesy American Physiological Society).*

Dill also confirmed that the lung was not adequate to maintain oxygenation of the blood during exercise at altitude, as Haldane had speculated on Pikes Peak and Barcroft had found in Peru. At sea level the lung alveoli are rich in oxygen, which easily crosses the lung membranes into the blood, and the blood oxygen level usually does not fall from rest to exercise. But at altitude, where the alveoli contain less oxygen, the large quantities required for exercise cross the lung membranes less easily and the blood oxygen level falls from rest to exercise. The lowlander's lung simply is not large enough to oxygenate the blood fully during exercise at altitude (West 1962). The high-altitude Andean natives have unusually large lungs, which contributes to their remarkable exercise prowess seen by Dill in 1935.

Dill used Henderson's famous equation to show for the first time the alkalinity of arterial blood at altitude. For the three men who went from Leadville to 14,000 feet on Mt. Elbert (fig. 5.2), the blood became even more alkaline. The hatchery men also had alkaline blood. With increased breathing at altitude, carbon dioxide, an acid, is blown off, and apparently the kidney, which is responsible for long-term acid-base balance, only partially restores the balance, even in lifelong residents. Haldane, from his measurements on Pikes Peak (chap. 2), had predicted this result, and Dill showed him to be correct.

Dill's group made the first measurements of blood lactate at high altitude. Many decades earlier, when yeast cells were deprived of oxygen, they could not burn glucose completely. The lactate that formed was considered a kind of waste product due to lack of oxygen. When Dill measured lactate in Leadville, for a given exercise workload the levels were higher in Leadville than in Boston, as he had expected. In recent years, although Dill's findings have been confirmed, their basis is hotly debated.

Because all of Dill's new findings led to new questions, new hypotheses, and new lines of research, one might say Dill caught new fish in Leadville. We suspect Barcroft came to rue his comment that altitude research was not worth doing below 14,000 feet.

For some sixty years after Leadville, Dill's interest in exercise and the environment resulted in scores of papers, books, and presentations. Where did Dill get his enthusiasm for exercise, and where for research? The Leadville study in 1929 and his suggestion to us in 1963 did not appear like water suddenly springing up in the desert. In Dill's case, college sports initiated his exercise interest, and it resurfaced when he became a high-school coach. Oddly the interest appeared again in 1918 in the Pacific Coast Fish Investigations (Dill 1921a, b). What was a trickle of exercise research became a stream in 1925 as it flowed through the Harvard Fatigue Laboratory and in 1929 when it flowed through the Leadville fish hatchery on the banks of the Arkansas River. The river of research became a torrent, subsequently flowing through the Andes of South America and the White Mountains of California. It is curious how the meandering of this stream proceeded from sport to research, fish to humans, Pacific to Atlantic, biochemistry to physiology, and sea level to high altitude. Let us follow this meandering.

As a student at Occidental College in California (fig. 5.5), Dill found that he had athletic ability and that he relished competition, particularly in track. He wrote, "I was on the track team for four years, captain in my junior year. The extraordinary event in my time was a defeat of USC [University of Southern California], I believe in 1911. A sports page from the Los Angeles paper [carried] the headline, 'If Dill beats Kelly, Oxy may win.' Not only did I beat Kelly in the high hurdles, every member of our team performed in record style." Later in 1914, while he was a graduate student for his M.A. in chemistry at Stanford, he competed against the undergraduates with a time of "53 seconds— as fast as I ever ran a quarter mile." In 1916, during his years of teaching, while he was the principal of the El Dorado County High School in Placerville, California, his interest in athletics surfaced again. "At the high school, administrative duties were trifling. I was busy teaching biology and physics and coaching girls' and boys' basketball and track. My good reputation at Placerville was based on turning out championship teams."

On April 6, 1917, the United States entered World War I. Through an odd series of events, the national crisis led Dill up a "fish ladder" to the physiology of exercise. As the war began to take its toll on the resources of the United States, a serious meat shortage developed. Being a chemist, Dill was enlisted by the Bureau of Chemistry into the U.S. Fish Commission as a specialist in fish investigations on the Pacific coast. As the fish canneries strove to compensate for the national meat shortage, Dill was to search for changes in the composition of fish and to provide technical advice to the canneries. Using a very simple strategy, he repeatedly took fish from the daily catch for chemical analysis. In sardines, for example, he found that protein content was rather constant at about 18 to 20 percent of the meat, month after month. But the fat content, which remained from 15 to 21 percent in December through March, plummeted suddenly to less than 1 percent in April, at which time the fish would be less palatable and less nutritious. How to explain this sudden loss of fat? He postulated that "the migration of schools may be related to the sudden decrease in fat content that takes place in April of each season." If so, the cause was exertion in cold water, where the fish were using fat as fuel for protracted exercise. Thus research in fish had focused his thinking on the combined effects of prolonged exercise and environment.

Such clear findings in the national interest at a time of crisis did not go unnoticed, and the research provided upward rungs for Dill's future career in exercise research. C. L. Alsberg, the chief of the Bureau of Chemistry, who had noticed Dill and his work on fish, opened doors for his young subordinate. In 1923 he obtained for Dill a fellowship for a Ph.D. degree at Stanford. Then in 1925, the oral examiners for Dill's Ph.D. degree, Alsberg, Franklin,[8] and Swain,[9] did more than pass their talented student. Happily Alsberg, who was a close friend and former colleague of the famous Harvard biochemist L. J. Henderson, secured for Dill a place as a postdoctoral fellow at Harvard with Henderson. Not to be outdone, Franklin, who was a friend of the chairman of the National Research Council, helped Dill get a fellowship to pay his salary. As Franklin later reported, the chairman had said, "If you have a student for whom you would tear your shirt, let us know." We can't say whether Franklin ruined a shirt, but we do know that Dill received the award. With his fish research leading to a position at Harvard and a fellowship stipend, Dill now had a ladder for his subsequent research career.

The ladder led Dill to the top, namely, to Harvard's L. J. Henderson, a remarkable biochemist of great intellect (Dill 1977). The Henderson-Hasselbach equation remains the foundation for understanding acid-base balance in the blood, and Henderson himself was a Renaissance scholar with broad interests, including the environment and human exercise. In 1920 he arranged for the Harvard medical graduate Arlie V. Bock to study with Barcroft in England and to go with Barcroft on the 1921–1922 high-altitude expedition to Peru.

When Bock returned, Henderson had him study the biochemical properties of blood during exercise. When Dill arrived in Boston in September of 1925, Henderson assigned him to work with Bock (Bock et al. 1928; Bock and Dill 1931). It was the perfect assignment. Because of Dill's long-standing interest in exercise, he took to its scientific study as a fish takes to water. With Bock, his mentor, he formed a "friendship which only grew stronger with the years" (Dill 1967, 1981). Indeed, as long as the Dills were in Boston, Bock was their family physician. While Henderson was certainly the intellectual leader of the group, Bock and Dill directed the work in the laboratory. The power within this team began to attract talented young men who wanted careers in science, such as Talbott and Edwards from the United States, Fölling from Norway, Oberg from Sweden, and Caulaert from France. News spread rapidly of important research from the laboratory, prompting the Nobel laureate A. V. Hill to pay a visit in 1927.

For Dill the great environment at Harvard soon got even better. In 1926 Henderson began to think of establishing a second laboratory to accommodate the increasing research activity and to give himself the office and secretary that Harvard had never provided. He negotiated for space in the semibasement of Harvard Business School's new Morgan Hall building and for substantial funding from the Rockefeller Foundation. Henderson saw a need for a systematic study of exercise and "what is vaguely called fatigue." So the Harvard Fatigue Laboratory received its name, and in the fall of 1927 Henderson chose Dill as the director (fig. 5.5).

As the director of the Fatigue Laboratory, Dill reported to Henderson. Even though Henderson's name rarely appeared on the papers that resulted, he closely followed the work of the laboratory, and he certainly approved of Dill's interest in maximal exercise and the "lack of oxygen and accumulation of lactic acid." In Leadville the studies of blood lactate and acid-base balance bore the stamp of Henderson's influence.

After Leadville, in Dill's long research career both at Harvard and after, he went from success to success. One might imagine he had all the resources that come from family wealth and powerful connections. Not so. He came from a poor farming family, was orphaned early in life, and some years after his first marriage went through divorce.[10] Somehow he rose to become a legend in American physiology, and in the

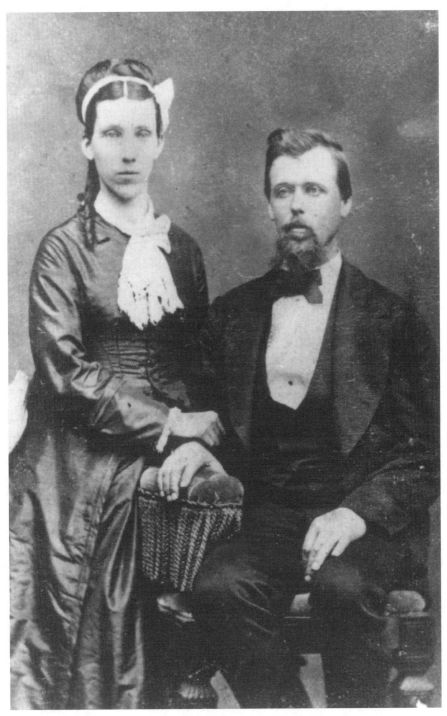

*Fig. 5.6. Wedding picture of David White Dill and Lydia Dunn, Iowa, 1875.
Photograph courtesy of David B. Dill Jr.*

years 1950–1951 became the twenty-third president of the prestigious American Physiological Society. What were the events in his family and his life that built the necessary character and motivation for such a distinguished career?

David Bruce Dill (1891–1986) came from a large, sturdy, and mobile family. His ancestors, the Francis Dill family, left Donegal, Ireland's most northwesterly county, in 1820 because life was so hard. Even in Ireland the Napoleonic Wars had adverse effects, causing a decline in trade and severe inflation. Landowners raised rents by dividing holdings into ever smaller plots, and the downtrodden Catholic majority (63 percent of the population in 1800) was threatening violence to obtain self-determination. The Dills were strong Protestants of the Calvinist tradition. Religious preference, economic hardship, and cultural instability caused the parents to leave Ireland with their six children, one of whom was Richard, Bruce's grandfather. America held promise, and the family settled near Kittanning in western Pennsylvania, where they engaged in farming and where in 1840 David White Dill, Bruce's father, was born. In 1866 he moved to Iowa where he met Lydia Dunn, who was also from western Pennsylvania. In 1875, when he was thirty-five and she was twenty-eight, they married (fig. 5.6) and settled in Wyman, Iowa. Although he was handsome and strong, life was not to be kind to him.

Mobility was in the Dill blood. The family had moved westward from Ireland to Pennsylvania, and from Pennsylvania to Iowa. Now, possibly in response to advertisements for settlers following the Civil War and the inducement of cheap land, much of the extended Dill family moved westward again from Wyman to Winchester in northeastern Kansas. In 1880 David and Lydia settled in a Covenanter Protestant community among relatives residing there since 1868. Hardly had they become settled on their new farm when some of the clan, including David and Lydia, moved westward again to Eskridge, Kansas, where there were more Covenanter relatives and more land. As it turned out, fortunately for young Bruce and his sisters some of the extended family remained in Wyman, Iowa.

Things initially went well for David and Lydia Dill in Eskridge, Kansas. The farm was productive; the Covenanter Church was active; there were other Dill and Dunn (Lydia's family) relatives nearby; and three more healthy children, including David Bruce Dill, who came to be known as "Bruce," were born. In 1890, although the Kansas farming economy had not been good for some three years, father David wanted horses and made the trip to Missouri, where he intended to buy a stallion. Instead of one stallion he bought two, and in order to make payment he unwisely mortgaged the family farm. Both stallions proved to be sterile. For a while these two errors—mortgaging the farm and buying worthless stallions—were tolerable. Then during Grover Cleveland's presidency came the Great Panic of April 1893, ushering in perhaps the most severe depression of the century and one destined to affect Kansas farmers for another five years. When, as was inevitable, the mortgage was foreclosed, the Dills lost their farm. Thanks only to the kindness and sympathy of Lydia's relatives, who owned a house, the Dill family continued to have a place to live, but their troubles were far from over.

Lydia became ill with tuberculosis, and in August of 1895 she died. Bruce was four years old, and his first memory is "walking beside the house in tears." Coincidentally, during the same year, most of the livestock on the farm also died of causes that were not known at the time but could also have been tuberculosis. After Lydia's death, the family was required to move, and father Dill found a cabin where they could live. Bruce recalls with gratitude the care and attention he received from his sisters after their mother died. Even though he was only four, they took him to school with them because there was no other way he could be looked after. Early one morning in 1896 the cabin in which they were living caught fire and burned to the ground, and although no one was hurt, nearly all their possessions were lost. David Dill was a kind man and a good father, but as a provider bad judgment and bad luck had caused him to fail.

The family was now totally destitute. In his memoirs Bruce wrote, "My father, with no resources but relatives, decided to call on them to look after his children. Three of us went back to father's sisters [in Wyman] . . . and it was my good fortune to be assigned to Aunt Rebecca [Aunt Becky and Uncle Lou Sampson]. My father hoped to bring us together again, but instead he died. . . . None of us saw him after we parted in 1896."

David Dill's obituary in the *Eskridge Star* of May 8, 1899, reads as follows: "Died: At the residence of C. R. Dill, Oakland, Kansas, Mr. David W. Dill, April 25, 1899, 10:30 P.M. Deceased had worked all day in the field plowing. He finished his day's work, ate supper as usual. Mr. S. F. Dill, who lives near him, a brother of the deceased was at the house visiting. The three brothers spent the evening pleasantly and retired about 10 o'clock. S. F. was awakened about 10:30 by the hard breathing of his brother. He attempted to awaken him, but could not."

Although sudden death from a heart attack was hardly known at that time, the newspaper account certainly points to that diagnosis. One wonders if chronic stress was part of the cause. The legendary sufferings of the biblical Job could hardly have been more severe than those of Bruce Dill's father, David.

For Bruce the move to the Sampson household proved a blessing, for Uncle Lou and Aunt Becky provided stability and opened doors of opportunity. "I came to realize there was great respect for Uncle Lou in the community. By my day he had been appointed director of two banks. . . . There was always [at the home] a monthly magazine, *The Atlantic*, a church paper, a farm paper and a Chicago newspaper. As soon as I could read I received the *Youth's Companion* with great pleasure." Once Aunt Becky told young Bruce, "My brother Dave, your father, was a poor businessman so you must learn what you can from Uncle Lou who is a successful businessman."

As a result of growing up with Uncle Lou and Aunt Becky, Bruce learned the philosophy of "waste not, want not," and, as shown by his Leadville expedition, he learned his lessons well. In 1929, if he were to go to the expense and trouble of mounting a substantial research expedition to Leadville, he wanted to have a number of scientific "fish to fry." His design of the project made obvious that he was testing numerous questions that involved concept and methodology, rest and exercise, breathing and circulation, chemistry and physiology, and altitude and sea level. By using the researchers as the subjects and by having prime laboratory space donated for the summer he did the whole project with little expense. Clearly Dill wanted to get his money's worth out of his efforts, and Uncle Lou would have been proud of him.

During the harsh Iowa winters in the early 1900s, Uncle Lou suffered much from asthma, and moving from the farm in Wyman to the city of Washington, Iowa, in 1903 didn't help. But when he made a visit to Cañon City, Colorado, his asthma improved, and he decided on a change of climate. Rather than to Cañon City, he moved the family to Santa Ana, California, where indeed his asthma disappeared. In 1904, when he built a substantial two-story house on a choice corner lot, the family settled in comfortably.

Being able to make friends easily, Bruce soon met Ben Blee, a neighbor his own age, who would be a lifelong friend. Ben's mother, he said, "became like a mother to me." When Bruce was a senior in high school, his girlfriend, Helen Austin, got typhoid fever, which required many weeks of convalescence. Bruce wrote, "I visited my friend the gardener at the Santa Fe RR. Hearing my need he cut a large armful of carnations of mixed colors. When Helen opened the door and heard my mumbled words, I could see tears in her eyes and heard a quiver in her voice as she thanked me." Not only did Bruce's thoughtfulness for others allow him to make many friends, but also he seemed never to forget those he made, for they popped up when most needed. In 1925, when his car broke down in Cheyenne, Wyoming, while the family was en route from California to Boston, he noted, "I didn't have enough cash to pay the garage bill. At the bank I found the teller had been one of my chemistry students of 1914–1916. We did some reminiscing and he cashed my check." Valuing friendship remained a lifelong trait. In 1935, en route to the Chilean Andes, Dill visited Carlos Mongé, South America's premier high-altitude expert, in Lima. Mongé was thrilled and commented how offended he had been when Barcroft had passed by in 1921 without stopping for a visit (Dill 1980).

Bruce's friendship with Ben Blee had its own rewards. In 1903 the school in Washington, Iowa, had advanced him one grade, and when he graduated from Santa Ana High School in 1908, he was one year ahead of Ben. As Bruce recalled, "Summer began with graduation and a proposal from Mrs. Blee that if I would delay entering Occidental College for a year, when Ben would graduate, she would make a home for both of us near the campus." Bruce readily agreed. Not only did the year off from school allow him the experience of being a foreman on a New Mexico ranch, but it also yielded earnings of $350 for college. When Bruce went to Occidental College in September of 1909, he found that Mrs. Blee was as good as her word and had indeed found a small cottage with a room each for Ben and himself.

Even if housing was free, $350 was not enough for college, and Bruce was concerned how he would manage. Somehow he had not grasped Uncle Lou's commitment to him, but it was soon to be demonstrated. While working on the ranch, Bruce had watched a solar eclipse through a poorly smoked glass and had sustained a retinal burn with loss of central vision in one eye. On arrival at Occidental College he told Mrs. Blee about the incident. She arranged for him to see an ophthalmologist, who said the injury was permanent and without remedy. Feeling his college career was doomed, Bruce returned home to get Uncle Lou's advice. Bruce reported, "I was surprised when he scoffed at my fears, emphasized that I had one good eye and that the defect was a minor matter. I think he guessed correctly that I had been discouraged by the spiraling cost I had been facing. Out of the blue he gave me a check for 50 dollars and told me to let him know when I needed more money. Convinced that he was solidly behind me in my desire for an education, I headed back to Los Angeles the next morning."

Not only did Uncle Lou care for Bruce's welfare, but Aunt Becky too was his strong supporter, although this had not been so apparent to him. In the summer of 1913 after his graduation from Occidental College she became very ill with cancer. In September, as he was leaving to obtain his M.A. in chemistry from Stanford, he went to Aunt Becky's bedside, and she "with tears in her eyes said, 'Good-bye Bruce Darling.' I guess pent-up love for me for the first time found expression. She died soon after." He was fortunate to see her true feelings before it was too late.

Uncle Lou lived for ten more years. He had the pleasure of seeing Bruce's marriage to Olive Cassel in 1913, Bruce's graduation from Stanford with a master's degree in chemistry in 1914, his success in high-school teaching in Salt Lake City from 1914 to 1916, his teaching, coaching, and job as a principal in Placerville, California, in 1916–1917, and his teaching in Palo Alto in 1917–1918. He saw Bruce's advancement with the Bureau of Chemistry during and after the war and had the pleasure of being a "grandfather" after Elizabeth (Betty) Cassel (1916) and I, David Bruce Jr. (1919), were born. He also knew Bruce was admitted to Stanford (1923) for his Ph.D. degree and had a fellowship to support his study there. He must have been gratified how handsomely Aunt Becky's and his investment of time, love, and money had paid dividends. When he died of kidney failure in 1923 in his eightieth year, he was living in Los Angeles with his son, Arthur. Dill wrote, "He left me 1,000 dollars, his Dodge, and many happy memories."

Dill received his Ph.D. from Stanford in 1925 and drove and camped with his family across the country to the East Coast, visiting relatives along the way. His arrival at Harvard University was not really a destination that September, but the beginning of a distinguished career. What had made that career possible? Bruce was constitutionally endowed with health, energy, intellect, and a warm personality. But those traits were encouraged to flourish because he received from earliest childhood the love and support of his family, particularly from Aunt Becky and Uncle Lou Samson.

In 1916, while Bruce and Olive Cassel Dill were in Placerville, their first child, Elizabeth (Betty) Cassel Dill, was born. Betty graduated from Simmons College, Boston, and while training as a nursing supervisor at Children's Hospital in Boston she became greatly concerned with the emotional problems facing children. This led to her obtaining her M.S. degree in psychiatric social work. In 1939 Steven M. Horvath (1911–) came from Ohio to Boston to work for his Ph.D. degree at Harvard in the Fatigue Laboratory with Dill. Betty and Steve met and in 1940 they were married. With the advent of World War II, Steve was assigned to Fort Knox, Kentucky, to study the effect of environmental conditions on men in the armored divisions. Betty worked with black children in Louisville, Kentucky. Later she also worked extensively on the problems of aging populations. After her death in 1988 a scholarship pro-

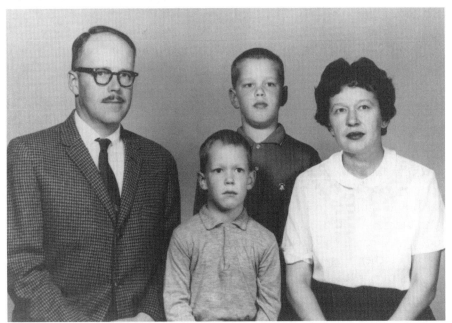

Fig. 5.7. David B. Dill Jr., his wife, Sonia (Lemish) Dill, and their two sons, Robin B. Dill (left) and Alexander C. Dill (right), November 1961. Photograph courtesy of David B. Dill Jr.

gram for minority students and a lectureship were established at the Simmons School of Social Work, and these were supported by the Elizabeth (Dill) Horvath Fund.

Steve Horvath went on to a distinguished scientific career, including founding in 1962 the University of California Institute for Environmental Stress at Santa Barbara, which he headed until his retirement at age eighty-five in 1997. He continues to do research, currently in diabetes and pituitary tumors at the Sansum Medical Research Institute in Santa Barbara. Steve and Betty Horvath published several books together, including the history of the Harvard Fatigue Laboratory (Horvath and Horvath 1973). The Horvaths' three children, Aletha, Steven Jr., and Peter, are all married, and each has two children. Aletha is a professor of psychology in the Virgin Islands, Steven Jr. is an anthropologist at the University of Arizona, and Peter, who has followed in his grandfather's footsteps, is an associate professor of physiology and nutrition at the State University of New York at Buffalo.

I, David B. Dill Jr., was born in 1919 in Los Angeles County near the San Pedro fish piers, where my father then worked. I have fond memories from childhood of the Harvard Fatigue Laboratory and particularly the 1929 Leadville study. My parents; my sister, Betty, thirteen; and I all came in the family car from Boston to Leadville, where we rented a house for the summer right in the middle of town and about two blocks off the main street, U.S. Highway 24. Dad wanted me to climb Mt. Elbert, where three of the research party were camped at 14,000 feet (fig. 5.2), and then to go right up to the top at 14,433 feet. The Leadville paper carried the headline "Boy from Sea Level Scales Mount Elbert in Record Time" and reported: "Young Dill started the ascent from Emerald Lake . . . and returned there just 6½ hours later. He was accompanied by his father who went to the summit of Elbert to get blood samples from a group of experimental scientists located in a tent there. 'An approaching thunderstorm hurried us along a bit and aided in shortening David's climbing time,' said Dr. Dill."

My father was habitually truthful, but when it came to improving a travel story, he didn't mind committing an omission or two. The fact is, I'd become exhausted short of the summit and my father had actually *carried* me on his back the last quarter of a mile or so.

After graduation from high school in Arlington, Massachusetts, near Boston, I attended Harvard and graduated in 1940. Rather than follow Dad into physiology, I became a mining geologist. I married Sonia Lemish, an artist, and we had two sons, both of whom are now married (fig. 5.7). Following my retirement from exploration geology and a year of consulting, I entered the graduate history program at the University of Arizona, completing the M.A. in 1987. Since then I have been researching and writing American history. Sonia died in 1993, and in 1996 I married Amy O. Johnson, a retired college dean. Regarding my two sons, Alex is a lawyer and bond analyst in New York, and Robin is a geotechnical engineer and a partner in a Boston firm. Both Robin and Alex have one child. At this writing Alex's son, James, is Bruce's only great-grandchild who continues the Dill name.

Quite in the Dill tradition, Bruce Sr. and Olive Cassel Dill have left a substantial family legacy—two children, five grandchildren, and eight great-grandchildren.

Final Word

Bruce Dill's long and distinguished career, including his years at the Harvard Fatigue Laboratory, his work with the military, his advice on the construction of Boulder Dam, his studies at the University of Indiana, his many years at Boulder City studying the effects of desert heat in humans and burros, his service to the American Physiological Society, has been reported in detail (Dill 1938, 1980; Horvath and Horvath

1973, 1987). Although he was reasonably fit, the aging Bruce began to have premonitions of death several months before it occurred. In January 1986 at his home in Boulder City, Nevada, Dad and I met and discussed his wishes in great detail. He wanted cremation, but he would have a marker in the Boulder City cemetery on which, after his name and dates, would be engraved the following: "His ashes were scattered along the desert walk beginning on the east side of the intersection of Highway 95 and the power line road." The desert walk was thus memorialized in honor of the many students and visiting scientists who had participated in hot-temperature experiments, and even in honor of the two beloved burros, Maud and Mabel, that had been so important in his desert research.

Bruce Dill was interested in exercise performance, whether it be at sea level, at altitude in Leadville and Chile, in the desert, or in the environment of old age. In a final tribute to the desert his last book, published when he was ninety-four, was titled *The Hot Life of Man and Beast*. As he went through life, he himself was a subject in nearly all of the experiments, and thus he became an expert on his own performance as he grew older. In April 1985, at age ninety-four, when he gave his final scientific paper before the American Physiological Society, he presented the progressive decline in his own maximum oxygen uptake with increasing age, his last measurement being at age ninety-three. He was certainly the oldest person to have such a measurement. The results showed a precipitous fall from age sixty-six to ninety-three. He extended the line down to an oxygen uptake virtually incompatible with exercise and perceptively commented with a wry smile, "Next year I may be dead."

The next year, in April 1986, in the presence of a standing ovation, the American Physiological Society presented to Dill, age ninety-five, the Ray G. Daggs Award (1986) in recognition of his distinguished service to the society and to the science of physiology (fig. 5.5). Dill thanked the committee, recalled his long and friendly association with Ray Daggs, and concluded with the words, "I thank Dr. Morgan and the members of the council for approving the award. This is a great society, of which I am very proud to be a member. Thank you, and God bless you all." Two months later, on June 18, 1986, Bruce Dill died, a physiologist to the end. With his daughter's assistance, he was in the process of writing his last book.

Colorado played a key role for Dill in his long life, for it was in Leadville that he developed his interest in altitude and environmental physiology, which became dominant interests in his subsequent career. Dill's long life is of more than passing interest to Colorado. Quite in addition to his important scientific contributions from his 1929 study, his was the first of a long and continuing line of medical studies by other scientists in Leadville. Subsequently Leadville became a natural laboratory for human adaptation to altitude, with studies by scientists from the University of Colorado and even from around the world. Dill was a part of that tradition.

◁Notes

1. Archibald V. Hill (1886–1977) was awarded the 1922 Nobel Prize for his work (with Meyerhof) on metabolism in muscle. When he visited Harvard's Fatigue Laboratory, he was the Royal Society's Fouleton Research Professor at University College, London, and his book *Muscular Activity* (1926) had been published. A reason for coming to Harvard was to ask Bock and Dill to write a third edition of the popular book *The Physiology of Muscular Exercise* (Bock and Dill 1931).

2. L. J. Henderson (1878–1942) was a professor of biological chemistry at Harvard from 1919 till his death. His books, *The Fitness of the Environment* (1913), *The Order of Nature* (1917), and *Blood* (1928), established him as a broad scholar of science. In Leadville in 1929, using the Henderson-Hasselbach equation, which is still a must for medical students and physicians, Dill calculated blood acid-base balance from the bicarbonate and carbon dioxide levels.

3. A. M. Pappenheimer Jr. (1908–1995) was a student protégé of L. J. Henderson. He was a colleague of Arthur Conant, who later became president of Harvard. In 1958 Pappenheimer became professor of biology and head tutor of the biological sciences program at Harvard. Following his widely acclaimed work on diphtheria toxin, he became a member of the National Academy of Sciences and president of the American Association of Immunologists. He gave two prestigious Harvey Lectures (personal note from J. R. Pappenheimer).

4. The other two recruits from sea level were Bramlett and Bowen, about whom we have no other information than the mention of their names in the published report.

5. Ancel Keys (1904–) was born in Colorado Springs and now lives in Minneapolis. Following the 1935 expedition to Chile, Keys worked in the field of nutrition and developed for the American forces in World War II the famous K rations, where K stood for "Keys." As a pioneer in cardiovascular epidemiology, he documented the link between diet and heart disease, which led to his picture on the cover of *Time Magazine* in 1961 (source: Henry Blackburn).

6. August Krogh (1874–1949) and his wife, Marie, were Danish scientists famous for their contributions to the role of oxygen in biology and for their research in circulation. In their laboratory in Copenhagen many young people, including E. H. Christensen and Ancel Keys, were trained. August received the Nobel Prize for his work on capillaries in 1920.

7. Joseph Barcroft (1872–1947), a brilliant British physiologist at Cambridge University, was a pioneer in showing how blood facilitated oxygen and carbon dioxide transport; he may be considered the father of fetal physiology.

8. Edward C. Franklin (1862–1937), Ph.D., was a professor of organic chemistry at Stanford and a member of the National Academy of Sciences. He was recognized for his work in liquid ammonia. Although never taught by Franklin, Dill consulted him for advice, and they were good friends.

9. Robert E. Swain (1875–1961) was a professor, then chairman, of the Department of Physiological Chemistry at Stanford and later became president of the university. In 1913, when he was in the master's program, Dill developed close ties with Swain.

10. Bruce Dill became engaged to Olive Cassel in 1912 during his junior year at Occidental College, and they were married the following year. In 1942 they were divorced. In 1946 Dill married Chloris Gillis, a union that lasted until his death in 1986.

6

SMALL BABIES AMONG BIG MOUNTAINS

John Lichty Solves a Colorado Mystery in Leadville

Lorna Grindlay Moore, Ph.D.

Lorna G. Moore writes of John (Jack) Lichty, the first full-time faculty
member of the University of Colorado Medical Center to do high-
altitude research. Although his research contributed to a revolution in
the care of newborns around the world and at all altitudes, the
contributions were slow to be appreciated. Why? Let Dr. Moore tell
the story. As an internationally famous anthropologist who has carried
on Lichty's work, she is well qualified to tell it and to show how that
work continues to yield dividends for the health of the newborn.

—THE EDITORS

A healthy baby is every parent's dream. Thus, preventing unnecessary
deaths in newborns is a universal goal. In the last fifty years many
events and persons have contributed to remarkable progress toward
achieving this goal. One series of important contributions began in what
might seem an unlikely place—Leadville, Colorado, at an altitude of
10,152 feet. There John A. Lichty Jr. (fig. 6.1) solved the mystery of
why babies born at high altitude were small (Lichty et al. 1955, 1957).
Even though the babies in Leadville were full term, they were small at
birth because they grew more slowly in their mother's womb. And possibly they grew more slowly because of the reduced amount of oxygen
at high altitude. Although everyone knew that babies not carried full
term and born prematurely were small, this was the first recognition
that babies could be small from growing too slowly in the womb, or, in
medical terms, in utero. As is so often true when one looks back on
medical discovery, the findings seem obvious, as in this instance, that
how fast a baby grows in utero is an important determinant of birth
weight. But for physicians working early in the twentieth century the

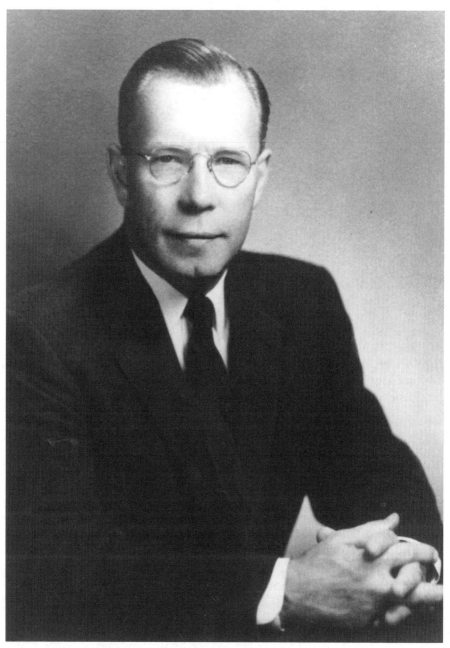

Fig. 6.1. John Alden Lichty Jr., ca 1952. Photograph courtesy of Roger H. Lichty.

focus was on prematurity, and slowed intrauterine growth was deliberately ignored. Yet a full understanding of what makes babies small is important because babies who are small at birth have a lower chance of survival, no matter whether they are born at high altitude or at sea level.

To translate his discovery into practice and to advance our knowledge about how oxygen is supplied to the unborn baby, others in Colorado, including Lula Lubchenco, Lichty's longtime colleague, and me, have continued the research. The insights that have been gained have ultimately led to practices that improve survival in newborns, not only in Colorado but also around the world. And physicians now identify, even in unborn infants, those who will need the greatest care. Current investigators who are working to learn how oxygen gets to the unborn and newborn child and how new treatments can improve the oxygen supply when it is inadequate are building on the foundation laid down by John Lichty.

To grasp the importance of Lichty's contributions in the late 1940s and early 1950s one must understand the times. Before and during the 1800s, neonatal mortality around the world was at least 20 to 50 percent of live births. From one to three of every five babies who were alive at birth died before they were one year old, primarily of diarrhea, pneumonia, or other infectious diseases. But by 1900 the germ theory of disease was being applied to public health; sanitation improved; water and milk were no longer contaminated; people understood the need for good personal hygiene; and infant mortality began to fall dramatically in the United States. As infectious disease killed fewer babies, other problems of the newborn increasingly became causes for concern, and prime among these was premature birth.

On the afternoon of June 7, 1935, the American Academy of Pediatrics convened at the Waldorf Astoria Hotel in New York City for a roundtable discussion on the problem of prematurity in newborns (1936). One of the notables participating, Dr. Edward Wagner of Cincinnati, reported his experience—when babies were born before the sixth month of pregnancy and weighed less than two pounds, they all died. If the pregnancies were one month longer and the babies were born one pound heavier, still only 30 percent of them lived. Even in the eighth month, for babies weighing less than four pounds, mortality was 38 percent. Dr. Ethyl Dunham of New Haven, Connecticut, commented, "Prematurity . . . is obviously the most important cause of infant mortality and a very high percentage of all the deaths take place in the first month [after birth]." Because of her concern that different birth criteria among maternity hospitals caused confusion in diagnosing "prematurity," she stated, "We have urged the use of 5 pounds 8 ounces [2500 gm] . . . if we can all agree on a [birth] weight to use [for diagnosis], it would be much easier to compare notes." Her recommendation carried the day, and the following resolution was passed: "For statistical purposes and comparison of results of care, a uniform standard for the diagnosis of prematurity is important. A premature infant is one who weighs 2500 gm or less at birth *regardless of the period of gestation*" (italics mine).

By disregarding the period of gestation (duration of pregnancy) the resolution had erred in promoting prematurity as the sole cause of low birth weight. Ignored was slow growth before birth, which could also cause babies to be small at birth. In retrospect the resolution seems strange in that the word "prematurity" itself implies only a shortened pregnancy, whereas birth weight even after a nine-month pregnancy could also be low if the baby grew too slowly in utero. Thus, babies could be small at birth because they were born too soon or they grew too slowly, or both. The causes of slow intrauterine growth often differ from the causes of early birth. Furthermore, as we shall see from Lubchenco's work (Lubchenco et al. 1972), these distinctions provided clues about infant mortality. The deliberate disregard of the period of gestation obscured the understanding of prematurity as well as growth rate in utero, and the incorrect definition impaired progress in the field.

Once errors are ensconced in the literature, they are difficult to eradicate. The error was expanded worldwide when the World Health Organization at its first assembly in 1948 defined "prematurity" solely as a birth weight of 5½ pounds (2,500 gm) or less (1949). In defense of the 1935 and 1948 resolutions it must be acknowledged that some uniform criterion was urgently needed for identifying babies at greatest risk. The 5½-pound threshold was simple, and information on the length of gestation was not uniformly collected, partly because physicians doubted that many mothers accurately recalled the first day of their last menstrual period. In 1961, some twenty-five years after the round-table discussion, health workers realized that a better definition was needed and made another attempt. "The Expert Committee on Maternal and Child Health of the World Health Organization has noted that the time has arrived for a reassessment of the international definition of prematurity and they have recommended 'the concept of *prematurity* in the definition should give way to *low birth weight*' " (Silverman 1963). Again, although this was a step in the right direction, simply to replace "prematurity" with "low birth weight" was not proper. Prematurity and low birth weight are not the same, and of course one does not want to discard the concept of prematurity.

Not until 1975 did the World Health Organization finally provide definitions of both prematurity and low birth weight. "Prematurity" was to designate babies who were born before the thirty-seventh week of gestation, where normal term was set at forty weeks. Babies weighing less than 5½ pounds (2,500 gm) were designated "low birth weight," even though the duration of pregnancy might be normal. At last, with this definition came official recognition that babies could grow too slowly in their mother's womb. Although it represented the flowering of an idea that stemmed from Lubchenco's work in the preceding decade, the 1975 definition had roots that went back to Lichty's studies in Leadville, Colorado, a quarter of a century earlier.

***

The Colorado story begins with Harry H. Gordon (1906–1988), who in 1946 came from Cornell University Medical School in New York City to be the first full-time chairman of the Department of Pediatrics at the University of Colorado School of Medicine in Denver. Since 1932 he had worked in the nursery for premature babies, and he had published some fifteen scientific articles, mostly on respiration and nutrition of the premature infant. Being in New York in 1935 and having as his primary responsibility the care of premature infants, he likely attended the roundtable discussion of the American Academy of Pediatrics and was attuned to the definition of prematurity based only on birth weight. Almost certainly, because of his expertise with premature infants, he was recruited to Colorado.

Because Colorado had the highest prematurity rate and the highest infant mortality in the United States, the state had an embarrassing problem, and the medical school knew it. With the end of World War II in 1945 servicemen were returning home from the military, and the country was entering the greatest baby boom in its history. Something had to be done and be done quickly. Gordon arrived in Denver and immediately began an energetic, regionwide assault on infant "prematurity" (Gordon and Lichty 1949). He established relationships with Alfred Washburn of the University of Colorado's Child Research Council, E. Stewart Taylor, chairman of Obstetrics and Gynecology, and persons at the Colorado State Department of Health, where he was given a joint appointment (Taylor and Gordon 1948). Gordon's vision was broad. With funding from the U.S. Children's Bureau, which Ethyl Dunham now headed in Washington, D.C., and with the cooperation of the several units from Colorado, he established the Premature Infant Teaching Unit in 1947. For the prevention, treatment, and follow-up care of

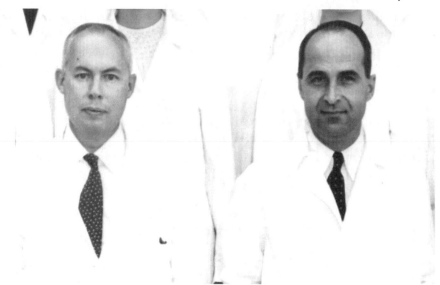

Fig. 6.2. Detail of a photograph of the obstetrics and gynecology department staff, 1955, showing Dr. Paul D. Bruns (left) and Dr. E. Stewart Taylor (right). Courtesy of Dr. E. Stewart Taylor.

"premature" infants he assembled an impressive team of pediatricians, obstetricians, nurses, nutritionists, social workers, and public health experts. It was a massive effort, and to direct it he recruited John A. Lichty Jr. An obstetrical colleague, Stewart Taylor (fig. 6.2), recalled those days. "John was very enthusiastic about the 'Preemie Project': he had brochures printed labeled 'Operation Preemie.' These were distributed to doctors and hospitals throughout the state" (1997).

In 1948, the first full year of the program, Gordon and Lichty reported on the state of affairs (1949), but they made no reference to the effects of altitude. Lubchenco notes, "Gordon was not aware of [the low birth weights in Leadville] when he came to Colorado" (1998). When the initial survey in Denver showed Colorado General Hospital had twice as many premature babies as occurred on the East Coast and Denver General Hospital had four times as many, Gordon felt, based on his previous experience in New York City, that poor nutrition and low socioeconomic status were the villains. He thought the same factors operated in Colorado, because Denver General Hospital, serving the poorer residents of the city, had the higher "prematurity" rate. Other factors he considered were ethnicity and inadequate medical care. He had overlooked Colorado's altitude; the state has the highest mean population altitude in the entire United States.

There was other evidence of the oversight—for when they established their Regional Treatment Centers, equipping each with an infant incubator, they excluded Colorado's highest city. Unfortunately their map of the state, showing where the incubators were placed, was published upside down (Gordon and Lichty 1949). Taking account of this error, one sees that only one of the eighteen incubators went to a town above 7,500 feet, and that was to Fairplay at 9,953 feet in Park County. Leadville, at a higher altitude (10,152 feet) and with a larger population, did not get an incubator. Gordon and Lichty had not considered altitude a factor.

However, another of their efforts proved to be far more important than they realized. They directed the Colorado Department of Health to revise the state's Certificate of Live Birth. Added at the bottom, for 1949, was a section that "*must* be filled out" and that included the baby's weight and length. Also to be entered was the "length of pregnancy," calculated from the first day of the mother's last menstrual period. Now for the first time in Colorado both the length of the mother's pregnancy and the infant's birth weight were available county by county for each child born in the state.

When the 1949 birth certificates began to come in, the information was dramatic. Of the 233 babies born above 10,000 feet in Lake County, 45 percent weighed less than 5½ pounds (Lichty et al. 1957). The "prematurity rate" in Lake County was ten times the national average! For the state as a whole, 10 percent of the infants, still double the normal rate, were "premature." Yet, the reported "length of pregnancy" was near the norm of forty weeks. Lichty, who by now was firmly in charge of the project, was incredulous. The next year, 1950, gave the same results—infants had low birth weight, but the mothers had a normal pregnancy. And the higher the altitude, the smaller were the newborns. Lichty was a "reserved and even straight-laced" man, but he became excited and "was not silent on his findings" (Lubchenco 1998). Now for the first time Lichty realized that he must take account of high altitude. He would not rest, Lubchenco commented, "until he got the data county by county and eventually hospital by hospital." He believed the place to start was where the problem was most severe, Lake County, Colorado.

Oddly, just when Lichty had exciting new findings, Gordon lost interest in the project. "Gordon never talked about altitude on rounds or in his papers" (Lubchenco 1998). In April 1951 he addressed the medical alumni at Cornell on how university pediatricians could help meet community health needs (Gordon 1951). Surely, identifying a problem as important as high infant mortality and working to solve it in a specific community, Leadville, Colorado, would have been a prime example for his presentation. Gordon mentioned Lichty as a new member of the department, but said nothing of his work in Leadville. By mid-1952 Gordon had left Colorado for a job at Johns Hopkins in Baltimore. As Lubchenco wrote, Lichty "was certainly the mover in the studies, for Harry Gordon was not around." An appointment at Johns Hopkins was a prestigious career move for Gordon, but why did he not maintain some interest in the project he had begun and about which he had been so enthusiastic only a few years before? Lichty was turning the project into high adventure, but somehow Gordon did not approve. With Gordon's departure, Lichty carried not only the problem of Colorado's low birth weights but also the responsibilities of chairman of the Department of Pediatrics.

If Lichty was to solve the mystery of small babies in Leadville, he would have to learn about the city: Leadville, at 10,000 feet the highest incorporated town in North America, is the county seat and population center for Lake County. It was founded in the mid-1800s and had become a burgeoning mining community. By the late 1800s it was the largest and most prosperous community in the state (Coquoz 1967) and home to individuals like H.A.W. Tabor, the wealthiest in the country. In the 1890s, when the United States went off the silver standard, Leadville and silver declined together. By 1950, Leadville had only six thousand residents. The people of Leadville and all of Lake County were served by a single medical facility, St. Vincent's Hospital, founded in 1878 by the Sisters of Charity of Leavenworth, Kansas. Hidden in these basic facts were important questions.

Was food or water contaminated in this still active mining community, and if so, would that affect birth weight? With a half century of economic decline, were public health, sanitation, medical care, and nutrition adequate? As the population declined, who remained behind to make up Leadville's ethnic mix? Were there other socioeconomic factors involved? In winter, when heavy snow made transport to the hospital difficult, did women elect early induction of labor to be assured of medical care? Were the reported birth weights wrong? These were questions that must be addressed to solve the mystery of why so many Leadville babies were born small.

With so many questions to be answered and with the department to run, Lichty needed help. Fortunately Dr. Paul D. Bruns (fig. 6.2), a member of the Department of Obstetrics and Gynecology with an appointment at the Health Department, joined the research project. Bruns had an interest in fetal health and was an early investigator of hyaline membrane disease in premature infants. Dr. Taylor, Bruns's departmental chairman, recalled: "Paul worked closely with John [Lichty]. For instance, he checked to see that low birth weight infants were not the result of elective [early] induction of labor."

Even with Bruns's help more information was needed than could be provided by birth certificates. Someone must go to Leadville to inspect the medical records at St. Vincent's Hospital and to interview both the mothers and their physicians. With $500 of unexpended grant funds, Lichty hired Dr. Rosalind Ting (fig. 6.3), a widowed Chinese pediatrician, to do the job. Dr. Ting had been educated in Shanghai and Beijing, but had left China in 1949 when the communists were consolidating their hold on the country. Soon after going to the University of Michigan to get a master's degree in public health, she was diagnosed with tuberculosis and sent for treatment to Denver's National Jewish Hospital, where she recovered quickly. In 1950, while in Denver, she married. After returning briefly to Ann Arbor to complete her degree, she rejoined her husband in Denver, where in October of 1951 their son was born. When Lichty offered her the job of research assistant, she accepted and began work in 1952. "Leadville," she wrote, "was my first working experience in the U.S. I cannot believe that I was so 'brave' to take that job, with a baby only a few months old and a husband who was a graduate student. The work excited me when the collected data began to show some fascinating patterns. My newly acquired knowledge in biostatistics was most helpful."

On a weekly basis she traveled to Leadville, crossing the Continental Divide twice, once at Loveland Pass at nearly 12,000 feet and a second time at Fremont Pass at more than 11,300 feet. Although those could be treacherous passes in winter, her trips were worthwhile, for she found a treasure trove of information. As her first step she examined for the years 1949–1951 the records of 577 babies born in St. Vincent's Hospital, those of 633 babies born in Denver at 5280 feet, and those of babies born at sea level in Los Angeles, California. The hospital records supported the findings from birth certificates—babies weighed less at high altitude. She then extended the observations to 1953 and added records from another high-altitude Colorado community, Cripple Creek, at 9508 feet. Again birth weights were low at high altitude.

Having established the presence of low birth weights, Lichty wondered if factors other than altitude might be responsible. He recruited Dr. Elizabeth Dyar (fig. 6.3), a nutritionist from Colorado State University. Together, Dyar and Ting examined maternal ethnicity, socioeconomic factors, and diet. When they compared the mothers in Lake County with those from lower Colorado locations, the frequency of Anglo— versus Spanish—surnames was the same, and there were no differences

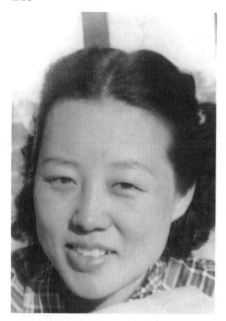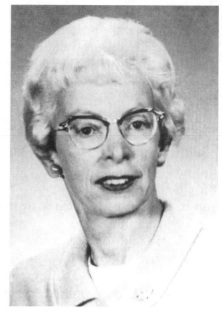

Fig. 6.3. Scientists participating in Leadville. At left *is Rosalind Ting, M.D., in the early 1950s. After working in Leadville, Dr. Ting passed her medical examination for licensure in the United States and in 1957, with Lichty's recommendation, joined the staff of the Children's Hospital of Philadelphia, where she has worked for more than forty years. She is now an associate professor emerita of pediatrics at the University of Pennsylvania. Courtesy of Dr. Rosalind Ting.* At right *is Elizabeth Dyar Gifford, Ph.D. (1912–1977), who from 1950 to 1976 was a dean at Colorado State University, Fort Collins, of what is now the College of Applied Human Sciences, housed in the Elizabeth Dyar Gifford Building. Photograph courtesy Colorado State University.*

relative to daily caloric, protein, trace mineral, or vitamin intake. When they performed chemical analyses of the water supplies in the various communities, they found no abnormalities. Using the tools available to them and being as careful as possible, Lichty, Ting, and Dyar concluded that high altitude was responsible for the low birth weights.

Maybe the birth weights were low because Leadville mothers were delivering prematurely and the birth certificates showing the normal "length of pregnancy" were wrong. Lichty wanted to verify whether physicians were accurately entering the gestational age. Because of her family responsibilities, Ting could not move there, but Lichty and Bruns recruited a young pediatrician, Dr. Robert Howard, who was just out of the service and was willing to move to Leadville for a year, taking his family in tow.

Howard attended 145 women through their pregnancies and deliveries. He confirmed the low birth weights in Lake County; babies weighed one-half to three-fourths of a pound less than in Denver (Howard et al. 1957a). For mothers who had given birth at low altitude and then again at Leadville, pregnancies were no shorter in Leadville, but their babies weighed less. From his careful menstrual histories of all the mothers, he found the pregnancies lasted thirty-nine weeks, the same as at sea level. In the few women who had induced labor in St. Vincent's Hospital, the duration of their pregnancies and the birth weights of their babies were the same as in women who had delivered spontaneously. Not only were the Leadville babies lighter in weight, they were also shorter in length and had smaller head circumferences. All these findings pointed to slower growth in the womb. The results were clear. Before birth babies in Lake County grew more slowly than at sea level, and this slowed growth—and not premature birth—caused Leadville babies to weigh less.

If altitude was retarding growth before birth, then the Leadville babies might not be getting as much oxygen as babies at sea level. Getting large quantities of oxygen across the placenta to a rapidly growing baby is a tricky problem even at sea level. In fact, the fetus must normally adapt to low-oxygen conditions, often referred to as "Mount Everest in utero" (Dawes 1967). Maybe the problem of getting oxygen to the baby was even trickier in Leadville than at low altitude because the air contained less oxygen. If Lichty could show that the oxygen level in the unborn child was less in Leadville than in Denver, he would have nearly "airtight" evidence that altitude had an effect on the unborn child. But how could he find out?

Haldane, on noting the bright red color when blood is highly oxygenated and the dark color when it is not, had suggested that the color of blood could be used to measure its oxygen level (chap. 2). An instrument that shined light through the skin to measure the color of blood in the ear had been developed, and Lichty used this new oximeter to estimate oxygen level in the ear when the head first appeared from the birth canal, but before the baby breathed (Howard et al. 1957b). In forty-nine Leadville babies, the oxygen level with a saturation of 50 percent was clearly lower than the 60 percent found in thirty-seven Denver babies. The measurements were made during, rather than before, birth, but the number of babies studied was large and the difference was great. Perhaps Lichty should have taken these findings more seriously, but he still was not convinced. He seemed to have been more impressed with how quickly and well the Leadville babies oxygenated their blood when they started breathing, as has been confirmed (Niermeyer et al. 1993).

Because persons going to altitude increase their number of red blood cells, Lichty thought the same process should operate before birth, but he didn't know that hemoglobin level and red cell count are not good indicators of oxygen level in the fetus. When he found no difference between Leadville and Denver babies, he felt he could not connect reduced oxygen in the womb to slow fetal growth in Leadville. He "was not one to say anything until he was sure of it" (Lubchenco 1998), but in this case he downplayed the low oxygen levels he had measured before birth in favor of less reliable evidence.

In his defense, such a study in humans was then, and is still, beset with difficulties, and it was several decades before definitive animal experiments confirmed that the fetus was actually hypoxic at high altitude. In 1968 Geoffrey Dawes, the famous English physiologist, commented on the "unsatisfactory state of affairs . . . where we cannot decide whether oxygen supply is likely to be a limiting factor to foetal growth." However, as more recent studies in fetal lambs show, despite compensations in both the pregnant ewe and the fetal lamb, the oxygen levels are still about 20 percent below sea-level values and account for the low birth weights of lambs delivered at high altitude (Jacobs et al. 1988). Over the decades, the work of Lichty and his colleagues has been vindicated by studies in human babies (Moore 1990). Subsequent studies in North and South America have repeatedly confirmed the slowed fetal growth in women living at altitude (fig. 6.4). Altitude slows fetal growth, and a lowered level of oxygen is the cause. Lichty's Leadville work, which established the existence of altitude-related fetal growth retardation, reflected his careful and thorough approach to research. His failure to emphasize low oxygen levels before birth in Leadville babies simply reflected his characteristically conservative scientific philosophy. Colorado's governor at the time was less cautious. "When John Lichty . . . announced the results of the study about low birth weight babies in Lake County, Governor Johnson commented, 'Everybody knows that gophers at high altitude are smaller than on the prairie'" (Taylor 1997).

As often happens, colleagues working on different problems come to learn their problems are not so different after all. By coincidence a longtime friend of Lichty's, Dr. Lula Lubchenco (fig. 6.5), was in the Department of Pediatrics but was part of a different group headed by Edith Boyd of the Child Research Council. While working on fetal growth for more than a decade in Denver, Lubchenco, with Drs. Charlotte Hansman and Marion Dressler, collected data from thousands of newborns. Year after year for babies born at term, birth weights were slightly less in Denver than in the United States as a whole, and a low

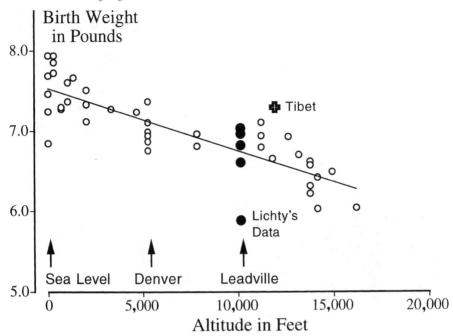

Fig. 6.4. *Fall in birth weights with increasing altitude, as reported from North and South America. Each circle represents a published value, and the line of best fit is shown. Filled circles show various studies from Leadville, Colorado, where more recent research shows improvement in birth weight since Lichty's report. Note the relatively high birth weight of babies born in the Tibetan population. Tibetans may have adapted so that in-utero growth rate is nearly the sea-level norm. Revised from Moore, 1990.*

socioeconomic class could not explain the difference. Lubchenco in Denver at 5280 feet and Lichty in Leadville at 10,150 feet had come to the same conclusion: babies grow more slowly in the womb when their mothers live at high altitude, and the higher the altitude the more their growth is slowed.

Not only did Lubchenco fully support Lichty, she went further. Because she and her colleagues knew both duration of pregnancy and birth weight in thousands of babies over a wide range of gestational ages, they could for the first time rather precisely calculate how fast a baby grows within its mother's womb (Lubchenco et al. 1963). There were great differences among pregnant women, and any of several factors, including altitude, could retard growth of the unborn child. When Edith Boyd saw Lubchenco's data, she went directly to the U.S. Children's Bureau in Washington, D.C., to get Dunham to change the

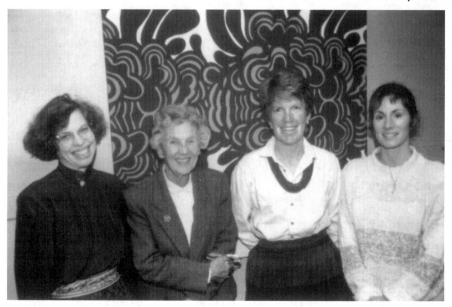

Fig. 6.5. Left to right: *Drs. Susan Niermeyer, Lula Lubchenco, Lorna Moore, and Stacy Zamudio in the late 1980s. Photo by Dr. Moore.*

definition of "prematurity" to include gestational age, but Dunham would have none of it.

Fortunately, the editor of the prestigious journal *Pediatrics* was more impressed. Upon receiving the manuscript of Lubchenco's 1963 article, he published it together with his editorial emphasizing how important the findings were (Silverman 1963). It was necessary to have these standards of fetal growth, he wrote, so that "aberrations can be identified." With some prescience, among the possible "aberrations" he mentioned, was the adverse effect of maternal smoking. The editor understood. He recognized fetal growth retardation could occur; that, when present, it must be recognized; and that the implications went far beyond mothers at altitude. Lubchenco and her colleagues continued their work for several more years to see which babies lived and which did not. In 1972 they showed the risks of growing slowly in utero. When babies grew slowly in the womb, they had higher mortality rates even when they were full term. Lubchenco had both validated and extended Lichty's work.

Entrenched beliefs are slow to change. Even though Harry Gordon had initiated the study of low-birth-weight babies in Colorado, for some reason he never acknowledged the key role of high altitude. Even by 1955, when the results from Leadville were clear, Gordon did not mention them in his paper on pediatric care of the newborn, although altitude-related complications of newborn care had wide implications for pediatricians. Why did Gordon mention neither Leadville nor Lichty's exciting findings from Leadville? After all, by training and experience it was Gordon, and not Lichty, who was the expert on the newborn. Perhaps Gordon's prior training led him in other directions, as Lubchenco implies: "He seemed more interested in relating low birth weight with social class, nutrition, and medical care [than to altitude]." Also, no published study had ever related birth weight to altitude. Elena Boder's personal letter suggesting a fall in birth weight with increasing altitude in Mexico was tucked away as a footnote in a 1952 yearbook article.

It seems strange that Gordon, who had put so much effort into the "prematurity" problem in Colorado and who had recruited Lichty, ignored the novel and important findings from his chosen lieutenant within his own department. Further, Gordon must have known Lichty well enough to appreciate what a careful, thoughtful, and thorough scientist Lichty was. Gordon was probably influenced by his years of training, his experience at sea level, and the concept of the 1935 resolution that small babies were premature. Indeed, the evidence suggests that he had his own preconceptions about "prematurity" and didn't believe Lichty's findings. One may speculate, but, in fact, the reasons for Gordon's silence on Lichty's work in Leadville remain a mystery. Whatever his reasons were, his reluctance to support, or even accept, Lichty's concept of slowed intrauterine growth at altitude surely contributed to the slow acceptance of this concept by the medical community. Even in 1998, when the Colorado State Department of Health was explaining why Colorado had the highest proportion of low-birth-weight infants in the United States, altitude was not mentioned.

———————◆———————

Who was this man whose discovery of altitude-associated fetal growth retardation was so slow to be accepted? First and foremost John A. Lichty Jr. (1906–1982) was a physician. With both his parents being physicians, he could hardly have escaped becoming one. His father, John A. Lichty Sr. (1866–1932), was an outstanding gastroenterologist at the University of Pittsburgh, president of the American Gastro-Enterological Association, vice-chairman of the American Medical Association, and vice-president of the American College of Physicians (fig. 6.6). He was also personal physician to the Pittsburgh financier Andrew Mellon.

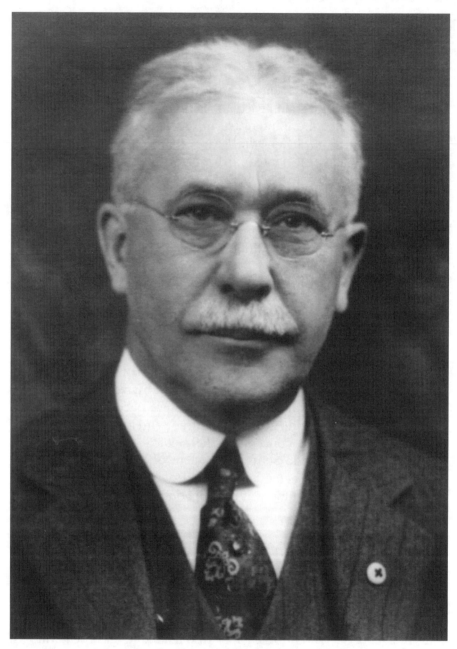

Fig. 6.6. John A. Lichty Sr., ca 1929. Courtesy of Roger H. Lichty.

John Lichty Jr.'s mother, Cora Stoner, and John Lichty Sr. had met in medical school. She was a remarkable woman. Although rare for women at that time, she specialized in internal medicine. While maintaining her own practice, she managed the practice of her busy husband, and somehow she found time to rear the four children (fig. 6.7) without a lot of help from him. With such a family background it is perhaps not surprising that John Lichty Jr. was destined not only for medicine, but also for achievement.

Born on May 30, 1906, in Pittsburgh, Pennsylvania, John Alden Lichty Jr. was the third child. After completing boarding school at Mercersburg Academy, he attended Princeton University, where he majored in biology and graduated *magna cum laude* in 1927. While still a medical student at the University of Rochester he worked in the laboratory of the famous gastrointestinal pathologist George H. Whipple, known for Whipple's disease of the gut. Together they submitted in January of 1932 three scientific papers (Havil et al. 1932a, b; Lichty et al. 1932), which because of the distinguished laboratory of origin must have been a source of great pride to young Lichty's father before he died in August of that year. Already as a medical student John A. Lichty Jr. was well on his way to a distinguished career in medical research.

After graduating in 1931, Lichty interned in medicine at New York Hospital in New York City. Because of his love for children, their attitudes toward their illnesses, and the quickness with which they healed, he chose to specialize in pediatrics. By emphasizing disease prevention a good pediatrician could contribute to his patient's health in adulthood (1951)—a concept that continues to gain importance. Although he began his pediatric training at Grace Memorial Hospital at Yale University, he returned to Rochester to complete it at Strong Memorial Hospital.

Probably because he had enjoyed working in Whipple's laboratory as a student, he chose a career in research, but now in the combined fields of bacteriology and immunology, rather than in gastroenterology. In those years acute rheumatic fever was common in children, and its sequel of rheumatic heart disease was devastating in adults. The question of the day was why acute rheumatic fever in children so often followed a "strep throat." When Lichty found antibodies against the streptococcus in the blood of rheumatic-fever patients, he helped build the link between the bacteria and the much-dreaded rheumatic heart disease (1941). It was very innovative work from a young assistant professor. The body's own immune response against the streptococcal bacteria damaged the heart valves. Lichty was a pioneer in show-

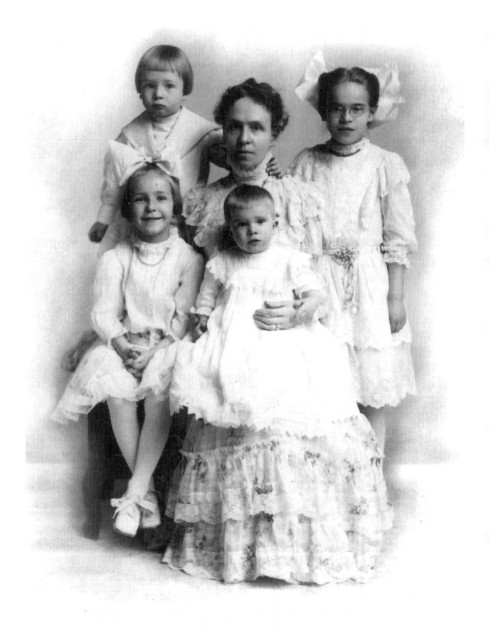

Fig. 6.7. Photograph of Dr. Cora Stoner Lichty and her children, ca 1910. Standing, left to right: *John A. Lichty Jr. and Dorothy Lichty (Lissfelt);* seated, left to right: *Marjorie Lichty (Hunter) and Joseph Stoner Lichty. Courtesy of Roger H. Lichty.*

ing that the body's immune defenses could cause an entirely different disease.

During World War II, when called for military service in 1943, he was first stationed in Pascagoula, Mississippi, and then, because of his expertise in bacteriology, he was sent to Camp Detrick, Maryland. There he did highly classified research on protection against bacteriological warfare, rising to the rank of lieutenant commander in the U.S. Navy. At the end of the war he returned to Strong Memorial Hospital to resume work on immune responses to infection.

Somehow, after three years of military service, he was not happy with his old position. He began to look toward public health, with its emphasis on disease prevention. Just before accepting a job in the U.S. Public Health Service in Washington, D.C., he met Dr. Harry Gordon, who offered him a faculty position in Colorado, with a half-time appointment in the Colorado State Department of Health. He would be working on the "Preemie Project"; after all, preventing the death of premature children was nearly the ultimate in preventive medicine. In 1947, after having visited Colorado only once, Lichty and Virginia, his wife of fifteen years, and their three small children moved to Denver (fig. 6.8). He was to spend the rest of his professional career in Colorado, a state that he loved for its climate and its mountains.

His love of the Colorado mountains was more aesthetic than scientific. After publication of the papers from Leadville he never pursued further questions relating to fetal growth retardation or to the effects of high altitude. In this failure to continue the work one wonders whether the resistance he sensed from Gordon and the lack of general acceptance of his findings were contributing factors. At any rate, his old desire to be more involved in public health surfaced again. In 1957 he took sabbatical leave from the University of Colorado School of Medicine and obtained a master's degree in public health from the University of Pittsburgh, graduating first in his class at the age of fifty-one. After returning to Denver, he resumed his position as head of the Division of Infectious Diseases at the Colorado Department of Public Health and his faculty appointment at the medical school. For the remainder of his career he devoted himself to studies of the immune responses to infections, rheumatic heart disorders, and the public-health aspects of heart disease. At various times he served as president of the Western Branch of the American Public Health Association, the Colorado Heart Association, and the Rocky Mountain Pediatric Association.

Both he and his wife, Virginia Harding, were active in the community. She was an accomplished cellist, who played in the Denver Brico Symphony and taught both piano and violoncello. Tragedy struck the

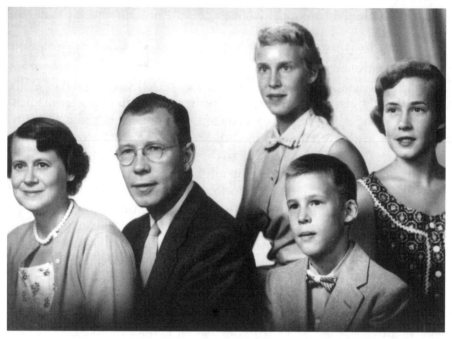

Fig. 6.8. Left to right: *Virginia H. Lichty, John A. Lichty Jr., Kathryn E. Lichty, Roger H. Lichty, and Priscilla Lichty (Moxley), ca 1956. Photograph courtesy of Roger H. Lichty.*

family in June of 1962 when the oldest of their three children, Kathryn, was killed in an automobile accident one week before she was to receive her master's degree in biology from the University of Colorado at Boulder and as she was preparing to enter the freshman class at the University of Colorado Medical School. One year later Lichty himself was diagnosed with Parkinson's disease. In 1968 he resigned his final career position as associate director of the Colorado Department of Public Health. He was one of the first Parkinson's disease patients in the United States to receive L-dopa, a drug that had not yet been approved by the federal Food and Drug Administration. Because the new treatment so successfully ameliorated his symptoms, he often volunteered to be observed as a Parkinson's patient in remission at medical conferences at the University Hospital. However, his nineteen-year battle with Parkinson's disease was one he ultimately could not win, and he died on February 1, 1982. Although a rather formal man, he was called "Jack" by those who knew him well. Lubchenco said, "Jack was one of the most honest persons I have ever known, and he gave credit to everyone." His longtime friend and minister, Alan Maruyama, said at the memorial service, "Jack Lichty was to me the epitome of what a doctor should be. He was gentle, kind, soft-spoken, wise, knowledgeable, patient, and merciful."

Virginia Harding Lichty suffered a massive stroke in 1984 and died from resulting complications on March 18, 1988. Her lifelong loyalty and support were major contributors to her husband's professional success, and her attentive care during his long illness probably lengthened his life and certainly made his final years more bearable.

Carrying on the Research: Author's Personal Note

Having long been interested in Lichty's studies of pregnancy and prenatal and neonatal life at high altitude, I have wanted to carry on studies in this field. In utero, where oxygen levels are marginal even under the best of circumstances, growth of the fetus is rapid, so nowhere is the effect of oxygen lack more important. Investigation in this area has been an exciting journey. In 1974 I came to Colorado as a postdoctoral fellow in the Cardiovascular Pulmonary Research Laboratory at the Medical Center, and it was there I began where Lichty had left off. Since not all babies born at high altitude were small, and if size at birth depended on oxygen availability within the womb, then, I reasoned, even at high altitude some mothers must be supplying their unborn babies with more oxygen than others. So, together with talented colleagues (fig. 6.5), I initiated studies in Leadville in the research laboratory established earlier by Dr. Grover (chap. 1) to see whether the amount of air a woman breathes and the oxygen levels in her arterial blood determine the size of her newborn.

As has long been known, women increase their breathing when they become pregnant. The increase has little effect on blood oxygen levels at sea level but becomes very important at high altitude (Moore et al. 1982a). In Leadville mothers who breathe more, arterial oxygen levels are higher, and they have larger babies than mothers who breathe less (1982b). But why do some pregnant women in Leadville increase their breathing more than others? We thought that some women were more sensitive than others to the low oxygen in the air. Oxygen in the blood is sensed by the carotid bodies, tiny organs about the size of a pinhead, located in the walls of the carotid arteries in the neck, and they send a signal to increase breathing when the blood oxygen level falls. Possibly some pregnant women at altitude had "sluggish" carotid bodies. To learn more, I went to Cerro de Pasco, Peru, at 14,000 feet. Because it is higher than Leadville, increases in breathing are even more important in maintaining blood oxygen levels (Moore et al. 1986). When women in Cerro de Pasco became pregnant, I found they increased their breathing nearly fourfold, far more than in Leadville. As in Leadville, some breathed more than others, and they gave birth to heavier babies. A mother's "drive to breathe," which is genetically controlled and originates in the carotid bodies, is one determinant of birth weight at high altitude.

But this wasn't the whole story. Even in pregnant women with big increases in breathing and relatively high blood oxygen levels, there was still a large variation in infant birth weight. We also knew that Tibetan women, who give birth to relatively large babies at high altitude (fig. 6.4), do not have a particularly large increase in breathing (Moore 1990). We had missed something, and we thought it might have to do with the blood flow to the pregnant uterus, since the amount of uterine blood flow is the key to a well-oxygenated fetus. In considering the problem, we recalled our earlier work in preeclampsia showing a strikingly increased incidence at high altitude in Colorado (Jensen and Moore 1997; Moore et al. 1982c). In preeclampsia the mother's blood pressure rises during pregnancy, and if not treated, leads to seizures and death. Because uterine blood flow is low in preeclampsia at sea level, we thought low uterine blood flow could be causing both low-birth-weight babies and an increased incidence of preeclampsia in Leadville.

Using ultrasound in Denver, we found during pregnancy increases in blood flow to the uterus of about 2 liters/minute, which is nearly one-third of the resting blood flow to the entire body (Palmer et al. 1992). But in Leadville blood flow increased much less (Zamudio et al. 1995a), and when there was preeclampsia, the blood flow was even smaller (Zamudio et al. 1995b). Mothers who pump more blood to the uterus have larger babies. When the baby does not receive enough oxygen to grow properly, it sends signals that increase the mother's blood pressure, in an apparent attempt to get more oxygen. But increasing the mother's blood pressure can threaten her own health. Clearly, at high altitude as well as at sea level, a high maternal blood flow to the uterus is the key to the baby's health and to the health of the mother. When Lichty found low-birth-weight babies in Leadville, he opened a new field of research, and that research continues today.

From sea level to the highest human habitation at nearly 16,000 feet, birth weight falls with increasing altitude (fig. 6.4). But avoiding small babies is not just about altitude. Pregnant women who smoke have small babies, as predicted in 1963 by the editor who reviewed Lubchenco's paper. Maternal smoking reduces birth weight by almost a half pound (Abel 1980; Meyer 1997). Smoking increases carbon monoxide in the blood, and this reduces the amount of oxygen the hemoglobin can carry (chap. 2). The more cigarettes a pregnant woman smokes, the greater her risk of having a small baby, and the risk is even greater if she smokes while living at altitude. Not only altitude and smoking, but other circumstances can reduce oxygen to the growing unborn baby as well. When the mother has heart or lung disease, which limits the oxygen supply to the baby, birth weight will fall (Novy et al. 1968; Shime et al. 1987). When the placenta, the organ of oxygen transfer from mother to baby, is abnormal, the baby's growth is retarded (Ounstead et al. 1985). During excessive exercise, the muscles can steal blood flow from the uterus. Healthy, physically fit women who do moderate exercise during pregnancy have normal-weight babies, but when nutrition or health is poor, even moderate exercise can lower birth weight by as much as a pound (Jovanovic et al. 1985; Lotgering et al. 1984). Possibly, as reported from Los Angeles, even air pollution can reduce oxygen delivery to the unborn child (Williams et al. 1977). Anything that inhibits normal oxygen transport to the fetus can retard fetal growth and put both mother and baby at risk. Lichty's studies in Leadville have implications for millions of people and go far beyond high altitude.

Lichty's were the first studies introducing both fetal growth rate and length of gestation as important for birth weight. Lubchenco followed with growth curves and risk of mortality. Others have added environmental and maternal factors affecting fetal growth and health, factors such as smoking, air pollution, exposure to toxic substances, congenital heart disease, sickle cell anemia, alcohol, and substance abuse. As one dedicated to public health, Lichty would have been pleased had he lived to see his impact on opening a field of medicine with enormous influence on the allocation of health-care resources.

The story has not ended. Continuing investigations at high altitude are helping identify how maternal oxygen transport determines fetal oxygenation and in turn fetal growth. Study of Andean and Tibetan populations, who have resided at high altitude for thousands of years, are providing insight into evolutionary adaptations. The specific finding of low birth weight at high altitude pointed scientists to the more general conclusion that both fetal and maternal well-being are affected by oxygen delivery to the unborn child. Methods not available to John Lichty now permit monitoring of fetal growth and the detection, and even correction, of developmental problems while in utero. John Lichty may never have fully understood the ramifications of his work in Leadville, which was but an isolated chapter in his life. However, because of that work, more parents can realize the goal of having born to them a healthy child.

7
WET LUNGS AT HIGH ALTITUDE

An Andean Problem Is Found in the Colorado Rockies

Robert F. Grover, M.D., Ph.D.

With extensive comments by

Charles S. Houston and Alex Drummond

How is it that Alex Drummond, who in 1958 was near an icy death from a mysterious disorder in the mountains high above Aspen, Colorado, has lived to tell his own story in these pages? And how was it that an Aspen family doctor, Charles Houston, played a key role in resolving some of the mystery in Drummond's disorder? Bob Grover, long a student of the disorder, with the help of the two principal actors puts this drama into perspective.

—JOHN T. REEVES

Deep within the lungs the branches of the respiratory tree divide into millions of tiny air sacs like bunches of grapes, called alveoli. Each alveolus wears a net of capillary blood vessels, and as we breathe, oxygen passes from these air sacs into the blood. Separating air from blood is a delicate layer of tissue, the alveolar-capillary membrane. This must be thin enough not to impede the transfer of oxygen, yet thick enough to prevent the leakage of fluid out of the blood vessels. As long as this delicate balance is maintained, the lung remains dry. However, if the function of this membrane is disrupted, the alveoli fill with fluid, blocking the entry of oxygen. As this fluid mixes with air, froth develops, gradually spreading up the airways and suffocating the individual. One literally drowns in one's own juices. This is pulmonary edema.

How does it feel to develop this life-threatening condition while struggling through deep snow over a remote, high mountain pass in the dead of winter far from civilization? Alex Drummond, a lad of twenty-one (fig. 7.1), knew how it felt. Alex and his companion, Pat, had decided to celebrate the entry of the new year 1959 by skiing cross-country from Aspen, Colorado, a small town in the Rocky Mountains at 7,800 feet, some ten miles up to frozen Maroon Lake at 10,000 feet, then over Buckskin Pass at 12,460 feet (fig. 7.2), down again to Snowmass Lake, and finally to ascend to the 14,092-foot summit of Snowmass Peak. They never made it. Here is what happened, recounted in Drummond's own words.

I shall never forget my good fortune at being plucked from the edge of an icy back country grave years ago. I think about it especially every New Year's Eve, for it was on New Year's Eve in 1958, one day before my 21st birthday, that I lay alone and wide-eyed in a dark tent in the Snowmass Wilderness wondering if help would come or if I would lie there and gradually fade away.

My adventure was simple and I am sure in many ways typical. I had flown from San Francisco to Denver on December 27th, met my roommate Pat, driven straight to Aspen, slept beside the car, then skied next day up the unplowed road past Maroon Lake and camped at the foot of Buckskin Pass [fig. 7.2]—comfortably but in below-zero temperatures.

Next day we crossed the 12,000-foot pass and today I shudder at the avalanche danger on that steep terrain. My poignantly clear recollection of climbing that pass is how colossally weak and irritable I was, especially irritable. Nothing was quite right, and in retrospect it was a warning that illness was on the way.

Skiing off the backside of the pass put us in no-man's land. Snowmass Peak, our 14,092 foot goal for the next day and for the trip, was almost touchably close, but the camera was frozen stiff and I could not record it.

That night I began to cough as my lungs started or continued filling with fluid. And the next morning I was too weak even to help pack up, leaving the toughest chore of winter camping exclusively to Pat. I was utterly exhausted, and could barely lift my pack onto my back. After doing so, I panted for several minutes to get my breath. With painful clarity I remember gasping for air, leaning over my poles and just standing there helplessly in the cold. It was not a panicky feeling of drowning, but of complete exhaustion and helplessness and groping and gasping and coughing.

There is something here that I think might be crucial for other parties, especially those composed of young and ambitious but inexperienced skiers. And that is that the victim's condition may not at first be taken seriously. It seemed implausible to Pat that I should deteriorate so quickly. It seemed like I was simply losing courage and therefore exaggerating a minor ailment.

Pat's suspicions were aroused because the very same thing had happened the year before when we had skied into Pearl Basin (~12,000 feet) above the ghost town of Ashcroft near Aspen. In exactly the same way I had grown ill and we had had to abandon the trip on the third

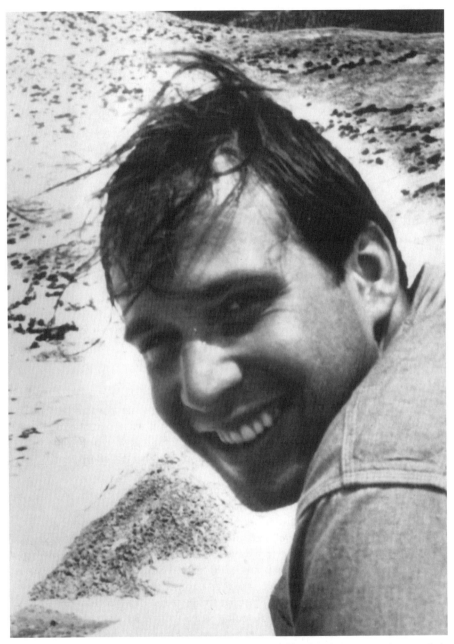

Fig. 7.1. Alex Drummond, who developed nearly fatal pulmonary edema while skiing at 12,000 feet over Buckskin Pass in midwinter, at age twenty-one. Photograph by Alex Drummond.

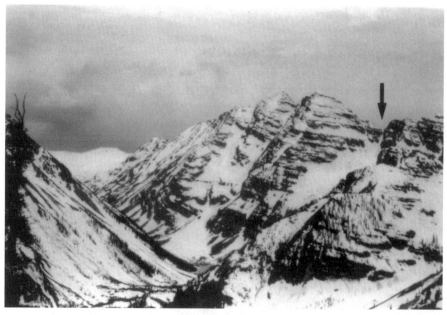

Fig. 7.2. Buckskin Pass (arrow), elevation 12,000 feet. Above and to the left *is North Maroon Peak, elevation 14,000 feet, towering 4,000 feet over frozen Maroon Lake* (lower left). *Photograph by Robert F. Grover.*

day, even though we had a cabin to stay in. That time it was all downhill for five miles to the car, and although it was an agonizing ski out because I was so weak and constantly falling, we got to the car, drove home (to Boulder), the condition quickly cleared up, and the whole thing was forgotten.

Even closer to this Buckskin Pass episode was a summer incident on Mt. Rainier about five months earlier in the summer of 1958. I manned a Park Service fire lookout at about 6,000 feet elevation, got moderate exercise doing chores and hauling water from a mile away, and spent most of my two free days each week climbing. In midsummer three of us camped at about 9,500 feet on Rainier's Winthrop Glacier to photograph the ice fall, then camped a second night in the summit crater at over 14,000 feet for the pure fun of it. Both nights were clear, calm and not terribly cold (probably mid 30°s). I slept under the stars while the other two slept in a tent. Emulating the technique of Bowery bums and one of my own Colorado heroes, I carried a Sunday newspaper and used wadded-up paper clumps as insulation to supplement my bag's warmth (I think I got a better bag before the Buckskin Pass trip in the winter). Much to my surprise, I coughed most of the second night and wondered what could be wrong. In the morning I felt like I had had a bad night but was not severely debilitated.

The difference from the other episodes may have been that the high altitude camping had not been preceded by a week at sea level, and hence the attack was less severe. In perfect weather we descended the normal route, losing altitude quickly and arriving at Paradise Lodge (5,557 feet) by noon. By then, all coughing had stopped.

Now it appeared that I was "ruining" another trip, and poor Pat was cross and disappointed and impatient. But to his great credit, he did everything necessary to help me. I raise the point because I have seen parties where a weak or sick member was blamed rather than helped, and in the case of pulmonary edema a back country party must turn its full attention to the victim.

Well, there we were, I could not possibly recross the high pass, and so we started slogging through loose, deep snow with 12 miles ahead of us to Snowmass Creek—the Snowmass resort didn't exist yet. However I was so debilitated that in a whole day of skiing we accomplished less than a mile. Standing more than moving, I frostbit my toes, but didn't yet know that.

Again we camped, and that night I raved—according to Pat—mostly about grocery stores. I don't know how even a 20-year old can think about food when what he needs to save his life is oxygen, but somehow my deranged mind conjured visions of grocery stores.

By morning I felt better and said I could go on. So we packed up and put on our skis, but had not gone more than a hundred feet when I collapsed. It was now clear that Pat would have to go for help. He put up the tent again and as I recall left both pads and bags, thus committing himself to having to make it to help before dark or face a night in the open without equipment. That was very brave and very risky but gave him great mobility.

After Pat left I remember lying there, feeling relatively calm and able to breathe tolerably well so long as I took rapid and shallow breaths and didn't do anything. Sometimes I looked out the tent door and saw that the world was still beautiful. Then came the long night alone, my most memorable New Year's Eve, wondering, "Where is Pat? Did he make it out? And will help come tomorrow?

Pat had, in fact, reached the Snowmass Falls Ranch and made contact by phone with a local family physician in Aspen, Dr. Charles S. Houston (fig. 7.3), who now takes up the story of Drummond's rescue.

Around seven o'clock that evening I was trying to clear my office desk for the New Year before going on to a dinner party. The phone rang: a young voice asked, "Are you the doctor? My friend is very sick. Can you come see him?" Pause. "He's camped up near Snowmass Lake. He couldn't go any further so I left him and came out for help." This was out of the ordinary even for a small-town doctor, and the other rescues I had gone out on were in the summer. I asked for details, and told the boy to hitch a ride up the valley and meet me at my home. Pat arrived two hours later and over food and drink told me the story.

As I heard the story it was obvious that the boy was in serious trouble and we would have to go in and carry him out. I assumed he had pneumonia and might not survive another night and day, so I began hustling help. There was no formal rescue agency in the county then; most rescues were done by volunteers who were themselves ardent climbers and skiers. But at nine o'clock on New Year's Eve I had trouble raising much enthusiasm and most of those I was able to reach told me to call again in the morning. The Sheriff volunteered his posse: "They're a great crowd, Doc. We'll go in there with the horses and get him out in no time at all." I was doubtful, knowing that the snow was soft and several feet deep. A call to the Army took time to sort out, but I finally got assurance that a helicopter would come over to Aspen at first light, and as a bona fide, a fuel truck would be dispatched at once.

But the bitterly cold weather was beginning to change, a storm was said to be coming, so I kept looking for a ground party, and finally, by midnight a group of seven agreed to meet at roadhead at dawn. Some one suggested that we get a vehicle to tow us part way in the interest of time, and after many inquiries I was told of a man who had a weasel, a small tracked vehicle that would carry four men and tow the others on skis. He would meet us at the end of the road at dawn.

Possibly I was the only one who felt well at 4:30 next morning, but at roadhead there was no driver and no weasel. An hour later he arrived, still angry because he had finally been found in bed with a woman not his wife and sparks had flown. But no matter, the weather was changing and rescue was hourly becoming more urgent. With the high wind and dubious weather there would be little chance that the helicopter could come (and in fact it did not). Some climbed aboard the weasel while others held to ropes and skied behind through the wilderness area which is now Snowmass Ski area and Snowmass Village, over a small pass and down to the valley. There the weasel had to stop. Pulling a toboggan belonging to my children, we skied up the valley alongside the frozen creek, Pat leading along the tracks he had made the day before. About noon we reached the little tent. Drummond was there, weak but alive, lying in his sleeping bag, head downhill. I carried him on my shoulders for the few feet to the toboggan, although every movement cost him a dreadfully exhausting cough. We bundled him in his sleeping bag and tied him securely on the toboggan. We started down about three o'clock, with wintry shadows already lengthening, dragging Drummond on the toboggan, of necessity head downwards, holding back on the steep places, and sweating hard [fig. 7.4]. The weasel was waiting for us, a welcome sight, and by nine o'clock that night Drummond was safely in bed in the old Pitkin County Hospital in Aspen.

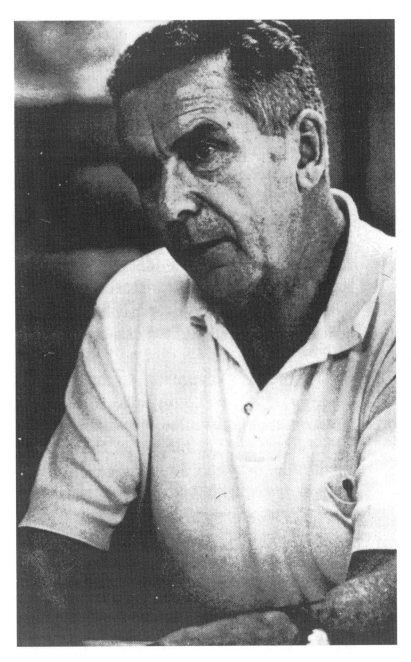

Fig. 7.3. Charles S. Houston, M.D., who organized and led the rescue party seeking Drummond on New Year's Day 1959. His publication of this case in a prominent medical journal was highly influential in alerting the medical and mountaineering communities throughout the world to pulmonary edema caused by ascent to high altitude. Photograph from Houston 1982.

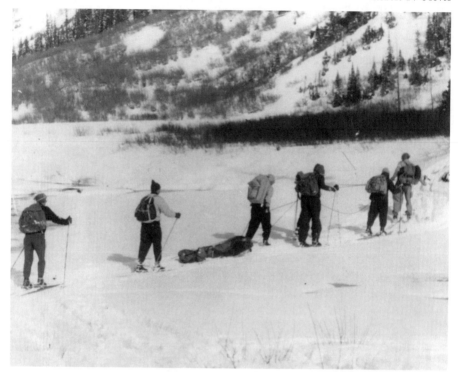

Fig. 7.4. Rescue party towing toboggan bearing Drummond. Members of the party were Ken Moore, Tommy Thomas, Dick Wright, Bill Mason, Marsh Barnard, Dick Durrance, Bill Craig, Pat Caywood (Drummond's companion), and Charles Houston. Photograph by Tommy Thomas, originally published in the Aspen Times, *January 8, 1959.*

On examination I heard many rales and wheezes throughout both lungs [noises heard through the stethoscope indicating fluid in the alveoli], and the X-ray showed patchy densities which could be broncho-pneumonia. The rest of his examination was normal, and he had no history of any significant illness. But it wasn't typical pneumonia: he had only a slight fever and his white blood count was only slightly el-evated. He immediately improved in the oxygen tent used in those days. Large doses of penicillin were started and I felt reasonably comfort-able with the diagnosis and treatment. I worried about his toes which were blackened with frostbite, as were the tip of his nose and his ears.

On January 8, 1959, the *Aspen Times* published photographs and a story of the rescue carrying the headline "Medical Data Gained from Ski Rescue Here": "A medical discovery of real importance to mountain-climbers may have been made here last week when a cross-country skier had to be brought out of the mountains by a group of Aspen skiers. . . . According to Dr. Charles Houston . . . it was first thought that [Drummond] was suffering from pneumonia. . . . However he said that he thought further study would prove that [Drummond], an athlete with a normal heart, suffered from a peculiar heart trouble connected with the altitude . . . and that the case would receive much attention from the medical world."

Unquestionably Houston had saved this young man's life. But from what illness had he saved him? The only thing obvious to Houston was that Drummond had suffered from fluid accumulation in his lungs (pulmonary edema). He wrote:

> The presumptive diagnosis was that the patient had bronchial pneumonia, but examination in the hospital showed that he had a temperature of 99.6°, a pulse of 96, respirations of 30. He was cyanotic [blue], and coughed almost constantly. His heart appeared to be normal in all respects and his blood pressure was 120/80. Both lungs were filled with moist rales throughout, more suspicious of heart failure than pneumonia. . . . The chest x-ray was interpreted by several radiologists as showing pulmonary edema, a type of congestion attributed to heart failure. . . . The chest x-ray cleared within 36 hours.
>
> This improvement was almost too fast for pneumonia, and I began to have second thoughts about the diagnosis. Examination had shown a normal heart with no murmurs, and with a normal blood pressure and no history of rheumatic fever (still common in that era), pulmonary edema due to heart failure seemed highly unlikely. But how else to explain the pulmonary edema? Next morning, I called his mother in San Francisco. She assured me that he had never had a serious illness in his life, did not smoke or drink and trained constantly; he seemed a totally fit and healthy young man.

Houston puzzled over the diagnosis for several months. If he was puzzled, he had plenty of company (table 7.1). North American physicians had not recognized this illness before and did not know what to make of it. The big question was whether or not Drummond had had heart failure. Below we describe the details of how the answer eventually came, but the chronology of events, table 1, summarizes how difficult the question was and how during the process of getting the answer opinions differed among some of the country's best physicians.

Even today the most common cause of pulmonary edema is heart failure. The main pumping chamber of the heart, the left ventricle, receives oxygenated blood from the lungs and pumps it throughout the body. When the left ventricle is unable to perform this pumping function (for whatever reason), then blood backs up into the lungs, blood pressure within the lungs rises, and fluid leaks out of the blood vessels into the air spaces. This is called cardiac (pulmonary) edema. There is nothing wrong with the lungs themselves. Rather, the lungs become involved as a consequence of a primary heart problem.

In 1959, when Houston rescued Drummond, conventional medical wisdom said that the second most common cause of fluid accumulation in the lungs was pneumonia (infection). However, the clinical picture including rapid recovery convinced Houston that Drummond had not suffered from pneumonia, and so he accepted the alternative diagnosis of heart failure. Formerly most respiratory deaths in previously healthy people going to high altitude had been attributed to pneumonia, so eliminating it was a major advance. Still he remained uneasy about giving Drummond's mother his diagnosis of heart failure in a young man with no known heart disease.

On February 16, 1959, just six weeks after the rescue of Drummond from Buckskin Pass, Houston received a very insightful letter from Drummond's mother. In retrospect, she is the very first one to put the finger on the correct diagnosis: "Knowing how he has exerted for years, I can't help feeling the explanation *must* be in the sudden change from mild sea level climate to extreme cold at very high altitudes, plus extreme exertion, naturally. These three episodes, it seems to me, cannot be just coincidence. Why has he not suffered this heart failure in high altitudes at other times when he has been living at 5,000 feet?"

What marvelous insight! There is not a great deal we have added in the ensuing years. Trust a mother to think the thing through in short order.

When Drummond returned to Aspen from Boulder a few weeks later, Houston tried to see if he could reproduce the "heart failure." After conducting all the appropriate preliminary tests he could, he had Drummond climb 4,000 feet to the summit of Ajax Mountain. At the end of that strenuous climb, Drummond felt fine. Nothing untoward had happened. Houston's examination indicated his lungs were completely dry. However, he thought he heard just a suspicion of a mitral murmur for the first time. (Blood flows from the lungs through the mitral valve into the left ventricle. Stenosis, i.e., narrowing of this valve, would obstruct blood flow and create back pressure in the lung.) On April 6, 1959, Houston wrote to Drummond's mother: "As a result of this I believe [Drummond] has mitral stenosis of a very minor degree, which is not apparent on routine examination. Under extreme conditions he develops pulmonary edema."

Fortunately for Drummond, time proved Houston to be wrong.

As Houston's prolonged struggle with the diagnosis continued, he sought the opinion of other medical specialists. He referred Drummond to the University of Colorado Medical Center in Denver in May 1959,

Table 7.1. Chronology of contradictory findings regarding the role of heart failure in high-altitude pulmonary edema (HAPE), 1958 to 1964

December 31, 1958	Drummond collapses in Snowmass Wilderness at about 12,000 feet
January 1, 1959	Houston leads Drummond rescue team
January 8, 1959	*Aspen Times* quotes Houston: Drummond had *acute heart failure*, not pneumonia
February 16, 1959	Drummond's mother claims that her son had *no heart failure*
April 6, 1959	Houston to Drummond's mother: he has a *bad heart valve*
May 1959	Drs. Blount and Mitchell: Drummond has a *normal heart*
May 22, 1959	Houston to Drummond's mother: Drummond had *heart failure*
August 1959	Review by Dr. Paul White: Drummond had *temporary heart failure*
October 1959	Houston submits report of Drummond's case to the *New England Journal of Medicine*
February 1960	Hultgren meets Houston and suggests they jointly write a paper on HAPE
March 18, 1960	Houston agrees to Hultgren's suggestion
March 1960	Hultgren and Spickard submit article to the *Stanford Medical Bulletin* on their medical experiences in Peru
April 1960	Houston's *Summit* article on Drummond: *probably heart failure*
May 1960	Hultgren and Spickard's article in the *Stanford Medical Bulletin*, a review of forty-one patient records in Peru: *probably no heart failure*
September 1960	Houston's article appears in the *New England Journal of Medicine*: *Drummond probably had heart failure*
April 7, 1961	Hultgren hears verbal report from Utah; Fred et al.: *no heart failure* in one HAPE patient
April 28, 1961	Hultgren receives prepublication proofs of his article (with Houston) in *Medicine*; does not incorporate findings from Utah
September 1961	Publication in *Medicine* by Hultgren, Houston et al.: *most likely heart failure*
Summers 1961/1962	Hultgren performs heart catheterizations in Peru
June 1962	Hultgren at Aspen conference reports his preliminary Peru findings: *no heart failure* in three HAPE patients
June 1962	Fred et al. publish article in *Circulation* about three Utah HAPE patients with *no heart failure*
March 1964	Hultgren et al. publish article in *Circulation* about four Peru HAPE patients with *no heart failure*

where he was examined by the chief of cardiology, S. Gilbert Blount Jr., together with the head chest physician, Roger Mitchell. By chance, the author (RFG) was also present at this examination. Blount reported: "There is no evidence upon which to base the diagnosis of any form of organic cardiovascular disease in this 21-year-old youth. It is considered that he has a normal cardiovascular system. Specifically, at this time there is no evidence whatever of mitral-valve disease. It is not clear exactly what happened last December."

Of course Drummond was also present. He recalls: "My vivid recollection is that in the darkened [fluoroscopy] room where Mitchell and Blount watched my heart in action, one turned to the other and said, 'Why, this young man has a perfectly normal heart.' . . . All I know as a layman is that I was pretty convinced, based on what I was told by you [Houston], Blount, and Mitchell, that my heart was OK."

Yet Houston remained unconvinced that Drummond's heart was not somehow involved in causing the pulmonary edema, and when he received Blount's report, he wrote to Drummond's mother on May 22, 1959: "Let me say once more—and you may read this to Drummond. Drummond definitely had congestive heart failure in December, and the cause was probably extreme exertion at high altitude under extreme conditions. Just what the contributions of work, cold and height were respectively, will not be known. He can go into failure again given the same or similar conditions."

Clearly Houston recognized that high altitude had contributed to Drummond's developing pulmonary edema, but it was not clear how. Nevertheless, he believed he should alert climbers and mountaineering physicians that apparently healthy individuals free of any heart disease could develop pulmonary edema while exercising at high altitude. Therefore, in the summer of 1959, Houston submitted an account of this case to the nonmedical mountaineering journal *Summit,* and the first published report appeared in April 1960 under the title "Pneumonia or Heart Failure?" In the discussion following his description of Drummond's case he wrote: "The best medical opinion which we have been able to obtain, in fact, the consensus of many opinions, is that this healthy young man without preceding heart disease went into heart failure because of the combination of strenuous exertion, extreme cold and moderate altitude. It seems quite possible that had the altitude been higher he might have died, and it is almost certain that failing the electrocardiogram and x-ray studies he would have been diagnosed as having bronchial pneumonia."

Later in 1959 Houston had the opportunity to have Drummond's case reviewed again, this time by the prominent Boston cardiologist Paul Dudley White. Houston had invited his old friend White, together with his wife, to visit his family in Aspen. He drove to Denver to pick up the Whites, and as they drove back through the mountains they talked about the case of Drummond and two similar episodes among mountaineers, so White was well briefed before seeing Drummond's X-rays and other data. As Houston commented, "Dr. White was then (and to my mind until his death) the foremost cardiologist in America, known and respected throughout the world. Before I went to K2 in 1953 I had consulted him and been reassured that my Himalayan climbing was 'a gigantic stress test' which proved I had no heart disease whatever. We had been good friends ever since. It was typical of Paul that when he walked in the lovely meadows near our home in Aspen he was joined by a number of his former patients—gardeners, musicians, participants in the Aspen Institute Seminars. They had heard he was in town and tagged devotedly behind the master on his morning walk."

After the two men had reviewed Drummond's case in private, White said, "Charlie, you must publish this case." On August 27, 1959, while the consultation was still fresh in his mind, Houston wrote to Drummond's mother: "Dr. Paul Dudley White visited me a few days ago, and spent some time reviewing Drummond's case and his cardiograms. He too was very puzzled, but finally felt that the most probable state of affairs was that Drummond did not have any heart disease but had had a temporary failure of the left ventricle causing his symptoms."

Thus the notion persisted that Drummond's heart didn't work well at high altitude. So, as suggested by Paul White, Houston prepared his now classic paper entitled "Acute Pulmonary Edema of High Altitude" and by October 1959 had submitted it to the prestigious *New England Journal of Medicine*; the publication appeared in September 1960.[1] The case of Drummond was presented in complete detail, together with brief accounts of four other cases in mountaineers. In his discussion, Houston speculates: "The mechanism of this type of pulmonary congestion is not clear. . . . Recent observations indicate that both acute and chronic anoxia [low oxygen] may cause striking elevation of pulmonary pressure, failure of the left ventricle and pulmonary edema. Since exercise and severe cold, together with anoxia, might have cumulative effects, this explanation appears to be the most probable."

The reader must bear in mind that at the beginning of the year 1960, physicians faced with a patient with pulmonary edema usually considered only two likely diagnoses, left heart failure and pneumonia. Virtually no physician outside Peru was aware that in the Andes a third possibility had been recognized (Bardáles 1955; Lizzárraga 1955). Rapid exposure to high altitude could result in acute pulmonary edema without left ventricular failure, a condition subsequently termed "high altitude pulmonary edema" (HAPE, or in England, where the spelling is oedema, HAPO). Hence, neither Houston nor the prominent physicians he had consulted can be faulted for not considering this third alternative.

At this point another player, the late Dr. Herbert N. Hultgren (fig. 7.5), came on the scene. Hultgren was a young cardiologist at Stanford University Medical School and, like Houston, an avid mountain climber. In February and March of 1959 Hultgren had the opportunity to visit

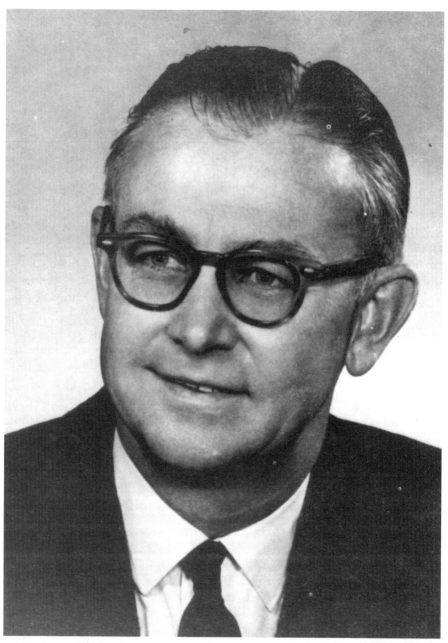

Fig. 7.5. Herbert N. Hultgren, M.D., at age fifty. Photo courtesy of Mrs. H. N. (Barbara) Hultgren.

Peru (as recently reviewed by Rennie 1999). He teamed up with his old climbing buddy, Dr. Warren Spickard, and together they spent two weeks at the Chulec General Hospital in La Oroyo at an altitude of 12,225 feet. There they were shown records and X-rays of forty-one patients with a condition known as *soroche agudo: edema agudo del pulmon*.[2] In all forty-one the condition had occurred within a few days of arrival from low altitude; nine of them had been ascending for the first time; the majority were high-altitude natives returning from a visit to the coast.

Hultgren wrote: "Although Soroche, acute mountain sickness [usually manifested by headache], is a well known phenomenon, little attention has been paid to the occurrence of acute pulmonary edema in some patients experiencing its discomforts. Only a few publications in Peruvian journals [in Spanish] describe this interesting complication of acute mountain sickness. The mechanism of this syndrome is unknown. The normal cardiac size and the absence of murmurs or gallop sounds during the acute stage suggest that left ventricular failure is absent."

This was a very significant observation because it indicated that HAPE, with its rapid recovery using only oxygen and bedrest, might be something other than cardiac edema. However, Hultgren and Spickard seem to have underestimated the significance of the material they had seen in Peru and chose to submit their observations to the obscure *Stanford Medical Bulletin* in March 1960; they were published in May 1960. Like Houston's first publication, this one too went virtually unnoticed by the medical community. For the record, however, this was the first detailed account of HAPE to appear in a medical journal in English.

Shortly before submitting these Peruvian observations for publication, Hultgren met Houston for the first time. Hultgren, who kept meticulous notes, wrote the author (RFG): "I found in my diary a visit to Salt Lake City for an altitude conference organized by Hans Hecht Feb 1960. There I met Charlie Houston. Here are my notes: 'Houston has a good collection of pulmonary edema cases from mountaineering journals and personal correspondence. . . . We should probably pool our cases and write them up as a separate report (Table 7.1).'"

On March 18, less than three weeks later, Hultgren received a letter from Houston saying "he will join us in the pulmonary edema paper."

Subsequently Houston added the following comment to his own paper being prepared for the *New England Journal of Medicine* (1960b), acknowledging this meeting with Hultgren: "More recently, Hultgren (personal communication) examined the records of a larger number of patients with pulmonary congestion believed to be due to acute exposure to high altitude."

It is unfortunate that he did not cite specifically Hultgren and Spickard's imminent publication in the *Stanford Medical Bulletin*, but apparently he was unaware of it.

Nonetheless Houston's paper in the *New England Journal of Medicine* was a landmark publication. His case report in English alerted physicians to a new concept, namely, that life-threatening congestion could develop following rapid ascent to moderate altitudes, even though the person was perfectly healthy at sea level. Furthermore, the rapid and complete clearing of the lungs following descent indicated that the congestion represented pulmonary edema rather than pneumonia, as had been suspected previously.

In real estate there is a saying that the three most important factors in selling a property are "location, location, location." One could say the same thing about publicizing a new medical discovery. Houston had selected the ideal location, the *New England Journal of Medicine*, for his succinct publication, which made a significant contribution to clinical medicine. Physicians in Peru recognized HAPE earlier, but history gives Houston due credit for generating widespread awareness of the existence of HAPE as a new concept in medicine.

Some years later Houston wrote: "My short article appeared in September 1960 and immediately attracted letters with similar stories from many countries. I was woefully naïve, unaware of suggestively similar reports in Spanish, published a few years earlier in South America."

Houston then goes on to review the earlier literature of which he was previously unaware:

> In 1955 Arturo Bardález Vega had described a few cases of "altitude edema" in *Anales de la Facultad de Medicina Lima* in Peru. Alberto Hurtado[3] had written a scholarly thesis for admission to the Peruvian Academy of Medicine in 1937. This was privately printed, and, like Bardález's 1955 paper, written in Spanish. Although this paper is widely cited, I know of no one who had read it until I had it translated at the University of Vermont. At least one of the five cases of altitude illness Hurtado described was probably HAPE. Then in 1983 I found a much earlier description, written in the third century by a Buddhist monk, about the death of a companion from HAPE on the Snowy Mountains of Central Asia! In May 1960, Herbert Hultgren and Warren Spickard had published in the *Stanford Medical Bulletin*, "Medical Experiences in Peru" (1960).

One year after the appearance of Houston's acclaimed case reports in the *New England Journal of Medicine* a comprehensive review of

HAPE was published in the journal *Medicine* written by Hultgren and Spickard, with Hellriegel, and Houston, as Houston put it, "graciously listed as co-author" (1961). This was a truly scholarly document containing detailed reports of fourteen cases Hultgren and Spickard had seen in Peru, complete with chest X-rays and electrocardiograms, and an additional thirteen cases Houston had collected from mountaineering literature. Included was an extensive discussion of four possible mechanisms leading to HAPE. After consideration of factors that could elevate the blood pressure in the pulmonary capillaries, Hultgren comes to the fourth potential mechanism, acute left ventricular failure: "This is of course the most likely cause of the syndrome. . . . The absence of consistent cardiac enlargement, the absence of other clinical signs of left ventricular failure and the absence of evidence of underlying heart disease, might suggest that acute left ventricular failure is not the *sole basis* for the pulmonary edema, and that other contributory factors are important."

This is a remarkable statement, for many cardiologists would interpret the absence of cardiac enlargement on X-ray as strong evidence against left heart failure. The authors acknowledge this paradox in their summary: "Although the most likely cause of the [pulmonary] edema is acute left ventricular failure, x-ray studies revealed no evidence of left ventricular or left atrial enlargement. . . . High altitude pulmonary edema appears to represent a unique effect of anoxia upon the circulation in man and deserves further study."

Hence Hultgren (who claims primary authorship of this paper) had reached the same conclusion set forth by Houston one year earlier. Or had he?

Events in Utah were unfolding that again led him away from considering heart failure. All that separates the air within the alveoli from the blood contained in the surrounding network of capillaries is a thin membrane made up of just two layers of cells, the wall of the capillary attached to the wall of the alveolus. If the pressure in the capillaries rises high enough, fluid is pushed from the blood into the alveolar air spaces, and the mechanisms keeping the lung dry can be overwhelmed. For example, if the left ventricle fails to pump all the blood it receives, the blood backs up into the lung. The pressure is raised in the left atrium, pulmonary veins, and capillaries. Such left heart failure is usually the first thought of a physician seeing a patient with pulmonary edema. The question of heart failure could be answered if left atrial pressure could be measured directly in a patient with HAPE. A high pressure would indicate heart failure and a low pressure would rule it out.

Fortuitously, left atrial pressure was measured during heart catheterization in a patient recovering from HAPE. In March 1961, the patient came to Alta, Utah, to ski at altitudes of 8,500 to 11,300 feet. On the second day he began having difficulty breathing (Fred et al. 1962). By morning of the third day he was desperately ill and was taken by car to a hospital in Salt Lake City (4,200 feet). The next day, March 29, while he was still recovering from HAPE, he underwent heart catheterization, which showed a high pressure in his pulmonary artery. However, by chance, the catheter pushed open an incompletely sealed flap in his heart and passed from the right atrium directly into the left atrium. The left atrial pressure was found to be *normal, not elevated!* There was no left heart failure.

As fate would have it, Hultgren first learned of these findings on April 7, 1961, barely one week after heart catheterization had been performed. A visiting cardiologist, Borys Surawicz, had just come through Salt Lake City en route to Stanford, where he included in his lecture the findings in Utah. Hultgren wrote in his diary: "This is amazing and I hope it is confirmed." Hultgren rarely used the word "amazing," so his excitement is obvious. The reader must realize that whether or not HAPE is a consequence of heart failure is a very important distinction. First of all, heart failure is not a diagnosis a physician makes casually, because the outlook is usually bad. Second, proper treatment depends upon accurate diagnosis. If heart failure is not the cause of HAPE, then treatment for heart failure is not indicated. Rather treatment should be directed at the derangement within the lung itself, as we shall see.

One can only conjecture about the events that followed. Three weeks after learning that physicians in Salt Lake City had definitely excluded left ventricular failure in HAPE, Hultgren received for final approval the printer's proofs of the paper (with Houston as coauthor) he had submitted to the journal *Medicine* some months earlier. The paper indicated left heart failure as "the most likely cause" of HAPE. At this point he could have, as is often done, inserted a "note added in proof" modifying his conclusion, based on these important new data. He elected not to; we shall never know his thinking.

At any rate, he and his colleagues returned to the Peruvian highlands in the summer of 1961 and again in 1962. While at the Chulec hospital in La Oroya at 12,300 feet, they performed heart catheterization on four patients suffering from HAPE, two of them on the day of admission. Their findings in all four confirmed those from Utah, namely, the pressure in the pulmonary artery was elevated, but there was no left heart failure. If anything, their data were even stronger than those from

Utah; they were collected before virtually any treatment, namely, without descent to a lower altitude and within hours of hospital admission.

In June 1962 Hultgren and Houston met again in Aspen at the first of the international conferences on pulmonary circulation, one of the now famous annual Aspen Lung Conferences. There was an all-star cast of both established and emerging investigators in the field. It was a great success. Houston chaired a panel discussion on the exciting new topic of HAPE, in which Hultgren, investigators from Peru, and a venerable physiologist from Minnesota, Maurice Visscher, participated. The published verbatim transcript of this session (Grover 1963) is a benchmark of the knowledge in the field at the time but is largely unread because unfortunately this publication again lacks that important ingredient, "location." Hultgren began with the autopsy findings from two fatal cases of HAPE, showing lung infection in one but not the other. Next he launched into an extended presentation of heart catheterizations he had performed on three patients with HAPE in Peru the previous summer. In the presentation, he said—completely without emphasis—"The pulmonary artery wedge pressures [indirect measures of left atrial pressure] were normal in each patient. . . . The data . . . do not support the concept that high altitude pulmonary edema is due to . . . left ventricular failure."

This was a major advance in HAPE, namely, that it was *not* caused by left heart failure. It was big news. Yet it was presented in such an understated fashion it went virtually unnoticed. In fact, Houston, the moderator of the session, only picked up on the question of the contributing role of infection. Not another word was said about heart failure. Incredible!

Another two years were to pass before the definitive publication of this information in March 1964, when Hultgren repeated this conclusion: "These data exclude acute left ventricular failure as a causative mechanism." Obviously Hultgren had reversed the belief he expressed in his paper in *Medicine* in 1961 that left ventricular failure was the most likely cause of HAPE. With this additional information, he was now convinced left heart failure was not the cause. The tortuous path leading to this conclusion is summarized in table 7.1. This is a prime example of the self-correcting capacity of medical science—but it does take time.

If a failing left ventricle is not raising pressure in the lung capillaries, could something else do it? Actually, yes, as suggested by a participant at the 1962 Aspen conference (Grover 1963) and later developed by Hultgren (1997). Forcing high blood flow through a small portion of lung will raise capillary pressure in that portion so high that fluid will leak into the alveoli. If, at high altitude, oxygen lack makes most of the small lung arteries constrict tightly, but a few don't constrict, then the lung artery pressure will rise and force too much blood through the areas of lung where the vessels remain open. The resulting leak causes collections of fluid, which appear white on the X-ray, sometimes making it look as though there were patches of cotton balls. The danger of combining high-altitude exposure with too much blood flow to the lung is dramatically seen in the occasional person who is born without a main artery to the right lung. The blood all goes to the left lung, which gets twice the normal flow. These persons seem perfectly healthy as long as they remain at sea level, but when they go to high altitude, they almost invariably develop edema, and it is only in the left lung. The great susceptibility of these persons to HAPE was first reported by Colorado researchers (Hackett et al. 1980), including the author. After thirty years the idea of too much blood flow to small lung areas (Hultgren 1997) is still deemed a plausible mechanism in HAPE.

Of course, if high lung artery pressure causes the fluid leak, the pressure has to increase before the leak can occur. Hultgren (with Colorado investigators, including the author; 1971) wanted to see if this was true. Recruited were five sturdy young men who were susceptible to HAPE, having recovered from one or more previous episodes. (Those who have had one episode are likely to have another when they go back to altitude.) Heart catheterization at sea level in California showed all five had normal pulmonary artery pressures, even when they exercised to increase blood flow through the lung. They then came to Leadville, vigorously climbed Mt. Massive—hardly an outing for tourists—and in the high-altitude laboratory in St. Vincent's Hospital had another heart catheterization. None of the five developed lung edema, but they all had very elevated pulmonary artery pressures. From this we inferred that the elevated pressure preceded the formation of pulmonary edema, rather than being a consequence of it.

If true, then preventing the pulmonary artery pressure from rising at altitude should prevent HAPE, and lowering pulmonary arterial pressure at altitude should be effective treatment. Both assumptions have since proven to be correct. A drug called nifedipine, which inhibits the pulmonary artery pressure rise at altitude, is now used both to treat and to prevent HAPE (Bärtsch 1991).

Does high pressure in the lung arteries and capillaries combined with oxygen lack at high altitude damage the thin membrane separating the air from the blood? There must be damage (Schoene et al. 1988; West 1994) because HAPE victims often cough up frothy, pink sputum containing very large protein molecules and even red cells that have escaped from the blood into the lung. There is also blood clotting within the lung, as was recently found (Hultgren et al. 1997) in lung tissue, which was remarkably well preserved, of two climbers who died from HAPE and were found sitting on a windswept slope high on Mt. McKinley—frozen solid! Thus in the forty years following Houston's publication, which led to widespread awareness of the existence of HAPE, we have learned a lot about it. Lung infection need not be present; the heart is not the villain; pressure is high in the lung arteries and probably also in the capillaries; there is damage to the thin lung membrane separating air and blood; and medicines that lower pressure are useful in both prevention and treatment. However, the initial cause and what makes some persons more susceptible than others remain mysterious.

Who is Charles Houston?

Charles Snead Houston began his life on August 24, 1913, in New York City. He enjoyed the benefit of an excellent education, graduating from Harvard University in 1935 and four years later from Columbia University School of Medicine. He was happily married to his wife, Dorcas, for fifty-eight years, until she died in 1999. Two major driving forces have directed his life: medicine and mountaineering. He has always loved taking care of patients. And he has viewed lofty peaks as a personal challenge since the age of twelve, when his father first took him to Chamonix in the French Alps to climb a small aiguille and in subsequent summers to many other Alpine peaks. In 1932 Brad Washburn, the world-renowned climber, mountain photographer, and author, took him to Mt. Crillon in Alaska, and in 1934 with a small party he made the first ascent of Mt. McKinley's neighboring peak, Mt. Foraker (17,280 feet). Then came even greater challenges as noted by Houston:

> In 1936, four of us at Harvard planned an expedition to Kanchenjunga, third highest peak in the world, elevation 28,146 feet. One of the four went to England to get equipment, and we invited four of the best British climbers to join us. . . . We had chosen to go to Kanchenjunga but fortunately the Brits persuaded Loomis (our emissary) that we weren't up to that and generously suggested Nanda Devi instead. Even when the first of us got to India we hoped for Kanchenjunga, but luckily we were refused. Nanda Devi (25,600 feet) was a great alternative and as it turned out, we made the first ascent of that mountain. The expedition was a classic. [Except when] one of the

members developed serious mental and emotional symptoms at our high camp, and I had to take him down, it could be seen as an example of what a great trip should be—and it was.

Two years later the American Alpine Club got permission to go to K2 (28,250 feet), the second highest mountain in the world, in the Karakoram Himalayas. They asked me to assemble a party "to find the best route for a *stronger* party the following year." We almost climbed it, halting just below 27,000 feet because of weather and running out of matches! Good climbers didn't push their luck in those days; mountaineering was a game.

Houston credits Ross McFarland, a pioneer in the young science of aviation medicine, with introducing him to the medical aspects of high altitude and also with leading him into the navy in September 1941, shortly before the Japanese attack on Pearl Harbor. He recalls:

In 1936, when I was 23, I met Dr. Ross McFarland. He had "taken me up" to 28,000 feet in a small tent-like room in which the percentage of oxygen was reduced slowly to one third (7%) that in sea-level air (21%). In the summer of 1941, WW II seemed inevitable. I applied for a commission in the Navy, and Ross McFarland introduced me to the Chief Flight Surgeon. . . . I got my wings a week before Pearl Harbor and was given charge of the high altitude training for aircrew at various places around the country during the next four years. Early in 1946, I was sent to Pensacola, Florida, where the decompression chambers offered an irresistible opportunity to answer that intriguing question: could Everest be climbed without supplemental oxygen? In 1924 on Mt. Everest, Colonel Norton had reached 28,000 feet. Could a well-acclimatized man go the small but deadly thousand feet higher to the summit and return undamaged?

The head of the Research Division of the Naval School of Aviation Medicine at Pensacola, Captain Ashton Grabiel, was immediately supportive. However, attracting scientists proved difficult. Joseph Lilienthal and Richard L. Riley had done the seminal work we needed, but Lilienthal thought the proposal was nonsense and refused to join. Riley, already one of the most distinguished physiologist-physicians to emerge from the accelerated experiences of the war, was more far-sighted, and we collected Frank Consolazio, John Selden, another flight surgeon Walter Jarvis, and a cardiologist John Patterson as helpers. I organized what came to be known [as] Operation Everest, while others (principally Riley and Consolazio) did the science. . . . But would the Navy approve what was likely to be a complex and difficult, and on the face of it, a rather risky task?

With approval from Washington in April of 1946 Houston and Riley proceeded to launch Operation Everest, in which one component of the mountain environment, hypoxia, was to be examined, using a decompression chamber (Sutton 1990). The objective was to simulate the profile of ascent of the world's highest mountain, Mt. Everest at 29,035 feet, with a barometric pressure of 253 mm Hg. Four men were sealed in the chamber, and over the next thirty days the chamber pressure was decreased progressively from 760 mm Hg (sea level) to 22,500 feet. Finally, with time running out, the investigators decided to "make a dash for the top." The chamber pressure was lowered steadily, simulating a climb of 1,000 feet per hour. At 28,000 feet, two of the subjects were given oxygen. The other two continued to breathe air right up to the simulated altitude of 30,000 feet, where they remained for twenty-one minutes. Although the two men remained fully conscious and well coordinated, they did not wish to attempt exercise or to go any higher. Houston had shown that humans could live breathing air on the summit of Mt. Everest and concluded, "My *mountaineering* goal had been accomplished." Some have sought cosmic significance in this juxtaposition of human and terrestrial limits. It is indeed remarkable that for the human inhabitants of earth the tolerable limit for low oxygen in the air does approximate the hypoxic challenge posed by earth's loftiest peak, the summit of Mt. Everest.

Following Operation Everest and after leaving the navy, Houston practiced medicine in Exeter, New Hampshire, as an internist, doing what was really family practice. In 1950, after a twelve-year hiatus in climbing due in part to World War II, Houston was invited to Lhasa with Lowell Thomas, the preeminent radio commentator, explorer, author, and journalist of the 1930s. When the communists got there first, Houston went instead with his father and Bill Tilman, the great British climber, to have a look at the south side of Mt. Everest. Hardly any European had ever crossed Nepal at that time, let alone seen that side of Everest. His enthusiasm for mountaineering thus rekindled, he organized a second American expedition to K2 in 1953, but they were hit with tragedy near the summit and barely survived. With a wife and three children at home, this narrow escape turned him away from mountaineering.

Robert H. Bates, Houston's climbing companion and close friend for some sixty-five years and coauthor with Houston of the book *K2: The Savage Mountain* (1955), provides insight into Houston's leadership style during his younger years:

> Charlie as a doctor is accustomed to telling people what to do about medical matters. If someone else has equal experience or more experience in a matter of debate he is never dogmatic. For instance on

K2 at one camp we were under the pressure of time to go higher next day. Two men thought that a big storm was imminent and decided not to go. The others went. The following day the weather had not changed and so the two who had stayed behind climbed higher and joined the others. However, that night a big storm struck. Charlie's decision had been made because of the number of days we were able to be on the mountain. Whether or not the weather would change quickly could not be determined. Some leaders could have been dogmatic and insisted that everyone leave at the same time, but Charlie did not. He realized that the opinion of the two who had stayed was based on experience as good as his own, and therefore he let them deal with the problem in another way. There were no hard feelings.

When we were highest on K2 in 1938 and again in 1953, although he was the leader of the expedition, he insisted each time that we have a secret ballot to see which two men would have the first and best chance to reach the summit. In life-and-death decisions Charlie thinks first and takes immediate control. He is a fine man when there are medical decisions to make or mountaineering decisions.

Charlie doesn't suffer fools gladly and he does not waste time. Sometimes he has dark moods when nothing seems to go right, but these don't last long and he returns to being his natural, cheerful, optimistic self.

In 1957 it was time for Houston to move on. He accepted an invitation to start a visionary program in preventive medicine in Aspen, Colorado, and he and his family moved there. The Aspen Clinic proved to be too far ahead of its time, and after eighteen months it collapsed, but by then Houston and his family did not have any other place to go, so they simply stayed and he went into private practice. But the quiet life of a small-town family doctor was not to last. His rescue of Drummond, the search for the cause of Drummond's illness, and the interest generated by it all may have prompted him to look for more adventure. He accepted an offer to become the director of the Peace Corps (1962–1966), first in India, then in Washington, D.C., where he acted as the director for Peace Corps volunteer doctors.

And then came a huge challenge. There had been in existence for some years the Icefield Ranges Research Project (IRRP), dedicated to scientific field studies in high mountain environments. How Houston became involved is recounted by Walter A. Wood, mountaineer, glaciologist, and geographer:

In 1966 the Advisory Committee of IRRP turned to me with an instruction to select a candidate to lead the yet-to-be born "Mt. Logan Study." No easier task could have come my way, for from more than thirty years of friendship and association with Charlie [Houston] in the fraternity of high mountain lovers, his distinction as a mountaineer going back to the 1930's set him apart for the task at hand.

A telephone call developed a spark of interest—a distinct plus when dealing with Charlie's characteristic caution—and this was followed by a meeting in New York, for which the trap had been baited with an irresistible cheese that Charlie promptly swallowed. From that October day in 1966, he gave much—if not most—of his professional and family life [for the next 14 years] to forwarding the Mt. Logan program. His leadership, his confidence and his convictions that carry the hallmark of conservative enthusiasm, all have combined to steer a scientific program to a safe anchorage. There were many times in those years when the very existence of the exercise hung by a thread or two, but so sure was Charlie's leadership and so dedicated were his lieutenants . . . [that this project] can now take its place as an inspiration not only to the medical fraternity but to the legions of lovers of the high places of the world. (Houston 1982)

Thus came into being the High Altitude Physiology Study (HAPS, 1967–1979), using the "real world" approach (Houston 1982). No simulation here: a laboratory, called Logan High, was constructed on a glacier at 17,500 feet on Mt. Logan in the Yukon Territory of Canada. Heavy annual snowfall over five years gradually buried the wooden laboratory constructed the first year under 40 feet of snow! New buildings were needed every few years (fig. 7.6). From 1967 until 1979, by virtue of heroic efforts, this facility was occupied seasonally by a series of investigators. Getting good scientists was hard, but they did come: Rennie, Sutton, Gray, Bryan, and others, some for a year, some for many. Obtaining funding was equally hard. It was a tough job, but it worked. Peter Hackett[4] also spent some time at Logan High, and from that started the Denali Research Station on a glacier at 14,000 feet on Mt. McKinley, where he, too, made major contributions to understanding HAPE during the next four or five years.

Selecting a remote glacier high on a stormy mountain proved to be the Achilles' heel of this project. Air support provided mostly by small fixed-wing aircraft was absolutely essential for delivering supplies and for transporting subjects and investigators to and from Logan High. And such flights required acceptable flying weather, which proved to be a rare commodity on Mt. Logan. For example, in 1979, the final year of this project, "the mountain flexed its muscles and bad weather prevented flights on twenty-two of the thirty project days. When weather was good the snow was unsafe for landing and takeoff" (Houston 1982).

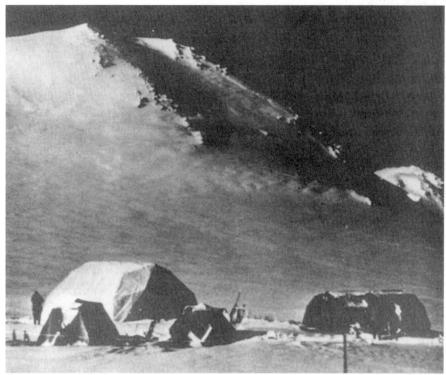

Fig. 7.6. Laboratory established by Houston on a glacier at 17,500 feet on Mt. Logan. The structures had to be replaced every few years as they became buried by the heavy annual snowfall. With support by aircraft, high-altitude research was conducted at Logan High, as it was known, for twelve years. Reprinted from D. Arnold, "Thin Air," Toronto Med. J. (May 1978): 105–109.

In a letter to Grover, Houston described an incident from the first year: "One member of the support party climbing up from 10,000 feet became exhausted and at 18,000 feet was unable to help himself. Storm delayed his evacuation, but thirty hours after reaching Logan High he was flown to Whitehorse, recovering remarkably on the way, though still unable to walk without staggering. He was found to have pulmonary edema, but recovered rapidly" (1999).

The precarious state of the personnel on Mt. Logan is vividly described in this anecdote:

> In 1969 a graphite pencil probably saved a life. A volunteer physiological subject flown directly to 17,500 feet from 2600 feet fell ill and lapsed into a coma. Oxygen was administered full strength but the subject showed little improvement. It was decided that evacuation

was necessary. As the radio was activated to call the aircraft, it blew a cathode resistor in the final amplifier stage. In those early days of the project we had no backup radio or spare parts, and we began to rack our brains for a substitute. Finally Casey had a thought: how about a pencil lead? The resistor is only 8 ohms. Out came an Eberhard-Faber wood pencil and we sharpened both ends and tested it. Perfect 8-ohms on the button! I soldered it into the set and we had a plane in a few hours. The subject recovered completely, beholden to a pencil that might have otherwise been used to complete some very important paperwork. (LaBelle 1972)

There were several near misses like this. Houston's task, as he saw it, was to keep the people as safe as possible, so he himself stayed mostly at Kluane base camp, talking twice a day by radio with the crew at Logan High; he flew up to Logan High only once or twice each summer "to show the flag." By 1971 the investigators "agreed that the risks of flying people directly to Logan High were not justified by the additional data obtainable."

More than forty research papers from Mt. Logan brought new information about high altitude, including descriptions of hemorrhages in the retina of the eye, altered kidney function, sleep disorder and its treatment, and premonitory signs of life-threatening brain edema. Houston collected the papers and reprinted them, together with a detailed description of the entire HAPS project. This volume was published in 1982 at his own expense and as of 1999 was still available.

Houston has often wondered whether the information obtained was worth the effort and expense involved. To put the research efforts on Mt. Logan in perspective, many investigations have been carried out in the "real world" of high mountain environments under less hazardous conditions. In 1961 the Himalayan Scientific and Mountaineering Expedition under the direction of L.G.C.E. Pugh erected a prefabricated laboratory ("Silver Hut") at 19,000 feet in the region of Mt. Everest, where sophisticated physiological experiments were carried out continuously for four months (Pugh 1962). As recently as 1998 Hornbein and his associates carried out research in a spectacular mountain setting in the Andes at the cosmic-ray facility at Chacaltaya, Bolivia, altitude 17,800 feet. Motorized vehicles can drive to this location from La Paz.

Houston's ultimate project, organized with John Sutton and Allen Cymerman, was Operation Everest II (OE II) in 1985, an expanded sequel to his first simulated ascent of Mt. Everest forty years earlier (Houston et al. 1991). During forty days six young men breathing air "climbed" to the summit of Mt. Everest in an altitude chamber at the U.S. Army Research Institute of Environmental Medicine, located in

Natick, Massachusetts, west of Boston. John Sutton, an altitude expert, physician, and physiologist from Canada, was the scientific leader and Allen Cymerman, head of the Altitude Division at Natick, was the facilities chairman, but Houston was the "commander." His was the supreme juggling act of keeping the subjects occupied, healthy, and happy in the chamber, assembling more than two dozen prima donna investigators, seeing to it that they accomplished their competing goals without coming to blows, and finding the money to do it all.

Throughout the conduct of OE II, both Houston and Jack Reeves kept personal diaries. In the publication from the project, Houston quotes extensively from both. Reeves provides some thoughtful insights into Houston's personality:

> . . . we are underfunded. I warned Charlie in the strongest possible terms about this drawback. . . . Charlie keeps the purse strings very tight . . . he lets no one in on the big picture. However, there are strongly positive sides to Charlie's leadership. . . . Most important is that through perseverance he has gotten the thing organized and is carrying it off. He has an instinctive judgment about human character which is nearly infallible. Thus, he has gathered a team of very good people which functions as a unit despite their diverse backgrounds. It works because of the quality of the people and also because Charlie sees that all activity flows through him. Thus, he keeps a tight control over logistical activities. Nothing has yet caused a major foul up in the machinery. He has done a good job of making tough decisions and of keeping everyone informed. Finally, he has the subjects' interests at heart. He is constantly present—he tends to the job and anything that is not going well, he is right there. The subjects sense this, of course, and they trust him. So, the tally card is strongly in Charlie's favor. It is remarkable that at 74 years he is pulling off so complicated an operation. One wonders what his wife thinks. And Charlie has said she is angry that he has not come home at least once: "but she has to get used to that." (Houston et al. 1991)

Houston's diary comments on some of these difficulties: "Indeed, the story of financing OE II is quite a tale in itself! Jack Reeves did in fact warn about this, but I had to go forward because the dates we could use the Natick decompression chamber were immutable. When the money did *not* come, I borrowed $25,000 on my own note to pay bills as they arrived" (Houston et al. 1991).

OE II was a great success. Measurements at heart catheterization, not possible on the real summit, were made on the simulated summit of Mt. Everest and showed, for example, that the resting pulmonary arterial pressure was slightly more than double the sea-level value and that the oxygen saturation in the arterial blood was about 60 percent of the sea-level value. At such great altitude the heart seemed to work very well even during maximal exercise, but the lung and brain functions were clearly impaired. Remarkably, the whole project went smoothly, a testament to Houston's organizational skills.

During the conduct of OE II, Houston was laying plans for yet another major field project, which was to study acute mountain sickness, not at 18,000 feet as on Mt. Logan but in tourists visiting the Keystone recreational area in Colorado at the more modest altitude of 9,300 feet, with ski lifts rising to over 11,000 feet. After the lifts and trails were built at Keystone, Bob Maynard, one of the founders, realized the need for an on-site medical clinic. Having known Houston for many years, Maynard asked him to set up a "model medical clinic" in Keystone. Houston accepted, planning began in 1976, and by the winter of 1978–1979, the Keystone Clinic had been established, with Houston in Vermont having an amiable arm's-length relationship. As the number of skiers in Colorado soared not only in Keystone but also in Vail, Copper Mountain, and Breckenridge, altitude illnesses became more common and pulmonary edema caused several needless deaths in healthy young people. In addition, although altitude headache was rarely life-threatening, it was far more common than pulmonary edema, and it caused a substantial loss of revenue for ski areas. Since Keystone is one of the higher ski areas in the Rockies, these problems were potentially serious. With prodding from Houston, the Keystone Clinic established in 1990 the Colorado Altitude Research Institute (CARI) to research altitude illnesses and to educate the public and the medical community about them. Although the Institute functioned well, it collapsed after three years for lack of funding. Houston's efforts to direct CARI "at arms-length" from Vermont also proved to be rather unsatisfactory. The Keystone Clinic itself was overtaken by the commercialization of medicine in 1993 when it was purchased by a health maintenance organization and became a "for-profit" outfit.

In 1966, Houston was appointed professor of community medicine at the University of Vermont, where he, now widowed, still lives. He has three children: Penny, who works as a counselor in California; David, who is a computer scientist at the University of Vermont; and Robin, a physician in Bozeman, Montana, who works under several contracts on infant nutritional deficiencies in third-world countries.

Houston has been made an honorary member of the American Alpine Club and most of the major mountaineering clubs around the world, including England and Japan. The King Albert Foundation selected Houston to be the recipient of its King Albert Medal of Merit for 1997, "a magnificent large gold medal." This foundation is an institution established in memory of the late Belgian king Albert I, who perished in a solo rock climb at Marche les Dames near Brussels in 1934.

Charles Houston is an organizer, a leader, a manager, a director; he is the man in charge. He organized and led major climbing expeditions; he directed the Peace Corps in India; he organized symposia on mountain medicine and the famous, still continuing Hypoxia Symposium in Canada; he conducted the Mt. Logan project; and he organized and directed Operation Everest and Operation Everest II. So, on New Year's Eve 1958 when Pat called, seeking help for his friend Drummond, alone and near death high in the frozen wilderness above Aspen, could Houston organize a rescue? Absolutely!

The Story Comes Full Circle

As for Alex Drummond, the opening character of this story, he wrote the following letter to Houston in 1991:

Before and since my HAPE episode life has been good to me. That same year [1959], I graduated from college, then studied for a year in Austria skiing and climbing in the Alps with all the ardor of a young man fulfilling a dream, and newly reassured that my heart was normal. Then followed several years as a nomadic Europhile, and a Masters degree in English at Berkeley where I gained political awareness during Berkeley's headiest political years. Then came my professional years, exactly twenty of them, in a satisfying career as Public Relations director for the National Center for Atmospheric Research in Boulder, Colorado—a time in which my two children, both good kids, grew from infants to adults.

At some point I could have tested myself at Himalayan or Andean altitudes but did not. Instead I loved more dearly the hills at home, learning from John Burroughs, the Hudson River naturalist: "That place is best loved which is best known." Home is now the whole West, with all its mountains, deserts, plateaus, and rivers. Exploring it has taken me across Colorado on skis along a 490-mile route that I carefully researched, twice across Yellowstone Park on skis, into the Canadian Rockies for a month of snow camping during the Calgary Olympics, and on annual spring pilgrimages to the desert canyon country. Regionalism is for me a philosophy and a practical activity. I belong to bioregionalism and Greens movements, lobby in the state legislature on regional environmental issues, and have written a biography of the Rocky Mountain naturalist, Enos Mills.

My mountain home (above Ward, Colorado, at 9,000 feet) is a haven from a troubled world for me and my frequent guests. It is simple, heated mostly by the sun, well supplied with books inside and flowers outside, and has electricity only once a week when I run a

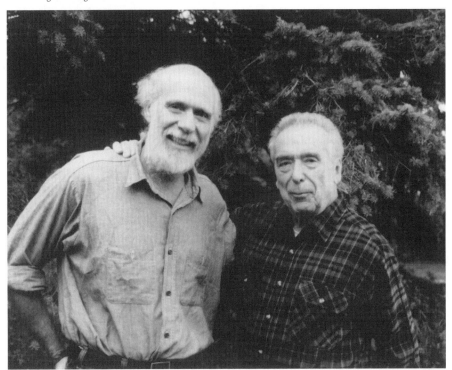

Fig. 7.7. Reunion of the rescuer, Houston (right), at age eighty-one, and the rescued, Drummond (left), at age fifty-six, years after the fateful episode of 1959. Photograph courtesy of C. S. Houston and Alex Drummond.

small generator. Of course I'll get photovoltaic panels when I can. More plans than I can enumerate still await me and I expect the good health which has blessed me since you [Houston] sent me home from Aspen Hospital to see me through many more happy years.

Is the susceptibility to HAPE passed from father to son? In 1990 Drummond wrote Houston, "When my son, age 18, developed gurgling noises in his chest on the third day of a backpack at timberline, we descended at once and the condition cleared up." If, indeed, the trait is inherited, then the genetics of HAPE are yet one other area of mystery in this most mysterious disease.

In 1994 Drummond visited Houston in Vermont, the first time they had met in thirty-five years, and they talked about the Aspen episode, which was still vivid in their memories (fig. 7.7). After this visit he wrote: "Let me say again how perfectly splendid it was to see you, and how much history in my own life, accumulated since that wintry day in 1959, added depth and meaning to our reunion."

Looking back on that fateful New Year's Eve of 1958, Drummond was indeed fortunate that his roommate, Pat, chose Houston as the person to lead the rescue. Possibly no one else in Aspen could have organized so effectively, from among New Year's revelers, a group of alpine skiers for a nighttime, winter mountain rescue. And few physicians would have recognized the unusual features of this isolated case and so doggedly pursued it to publication. Yes, a young man's life was saved, and sportspersons as well as physicians around the world were alerted to a new potential danger because of a high-altitude rescue in Colorado on New Year's Day 1959.

Notes

1. In the *New England Journal of Medicine* article Drummond is referred to as R. C. because his given name was Ron Cox. Sometime after 1959 he adopted his grandfather's name, Alex Drummond.
2. Translation: acute mountain sickness: acute pulmonary edema.
3. Alberto Hurtado (1901–1983), born in Lima, Peru, was a graduate of Harvard Medical School (1924) and had extensive postgraduate training in the United States. In addition to being a professor of the Faculty of Medicine in Lima and minister of health for Peru, he was the director of research for Instituto de Biología Andina, which is famous for high-altitude research.
4. Peter Hackett (1947–) is an emergency physician who established the Himalayan Rescue Association in Nepal, and who began and headed from 1981 to 1989 the medical research program Denali on the Denali Glacier on Mt. McKinley, Alaska. A premier climber, Hackett reached the summit of Mt. Everest in October 1981.

REFERENCES

Abel, E. L. Smoking during pregnancy: A review of effects on growth and development of offspring. *Hum. Biol.* 52 (1980): 593–625.

Alexander, A. F., and R. Jensen. Gross cardiac changes in cattle with high-mountain (brisket) disease and in experimental cattle maintained at high altitudes. *Am. J. Vet. Res.* 20 (1959): 680–689.

———. Pulmonary vascular pathology of bovine high mountain disease. *Am. J. Vet. Res.* 24 (1963): 1098–1111.

Alexander, A. F., D. H. Will, R. F. Grover, and J. T. Reeves. Pulmonary hypertension and right ventricular hypertrophy in cattle at high altitude. *Am. J. Vet. Res.* 21 (1960): 199–204.

American Academy of Pediatrics. Round-table discussion on prematurity. *J. Pediat.* 8 (1936): 104–121.

Anand, I. S., R. M. Malhotra, Y. Chandrashekhar, H. K. Bali, S. S. Chauhan, S. K. Jindal, R. K. Bhandari, and P. L. Wahi. Adult subacute mountain sickness: A syndrome of congestive heart failure in man at very high altitude. *Lancet* 335 (1990): 561–565.

Barazanji, K. W., M. Ramanathan, R. L. Johnson Jr., and C.C.W. Hsia. A modified rebreathing technique using an infrared gas analyzer. *J. Appl. Physiol.* 80 (1996): 1258–1262.

Barcroft, J., and E. K. Marshall Jr. Note on the effect of external temperature on the circulation of man. *J. Physiol.* 58 (1923): 145–156.

Bardáles, V. Edema pulmonar agudo por soroche grave. *Anal. Fac. Med.* (Lima) 38 (1955): 232–240.

Bärtsch, P., M. Maggiorini, M. Ritter, C. Noti, P. Vock, and O. Oelz. Prevention of high-altitude pulmonary edema by nifedipine. *New Engl. J. Med.* 325 (1991): 1284–1289.

Baumann, H., and A. Grollman. Über die theoretischen und praktischen Grundlagen und die klinische Zuverlässigkeit der Acetylenmethode zur Bestimmung des Minutenvolumens. *Zeit. für klin. Med.* 115 (1930): 41.

Bock, A. V., and D. B. Dill. *The physiology of muscular exercise.* London: Longmans, Green, 1931.

Bock, A. V., C. Caulaert, D. B. Dill, A. Fölling, and L. M. Hurxthal. Studies in muscular activity: Dynamic changes occurring in man at work, et seq. *J. Physiol.* (London) 66 (1928): 121–174.

Boycott, A. E., and J. S. Haldane. The effects of low atmospheric pressures on respiration. *J. Physiol.* 37 (1908): 355–377.

Boycott, A. E., G.C.C. Damant, and J. S. Haldane. The prevention of compressed-air illness. *J. Hygiene* 8 (1908), 342–443.

Cander, L., and R. E. Foster. Determination of pulmonary parenchymal tissue volume and pulmonary capillary blood flow in man. *J. Appl. Physiol.* 14 (1959): 541–551.

Chapman, C. B., H. L. Taylor, C. Borden, R. V. Ebert, and A. Keys. Simultaneous determinations of the resting arteriovenous oxygen difference by the acetylene and the direct Fick methods. *J. Clin. Invest.* 29 (1950): 651–659.

Christiansen, J., C. G. Douglas, and J. S. Haldane. The absorption and dissociation of carbon dioxide by human blood. *J. Physiol.* 48 (1914): 244–271.

Clark, R. *JBS: The life and works of J.B.S. Haldane.* Oxford: Oxford University Press, 1968.

Comroe, J. H., Jr. *Retrospectroscope: Insights into medical discovery.* Menlo Park, CA: Von Gher Press, 1977.

Coquoz, R. L. *The history of medicine in Leadville and Lake County, Colorado.* (Copy held by Colorado Historical Society.) 1967.

Cruz, J. C., J. T. Reeves, B. E. Russell, A. F. Alexander, and D. H. Will. Embryo transplanted calves: The pulmonary hypertensive trait is genetically transmitted. *Proc. Soc. Exp. Biol.* 164 (1980): 142–145.

Cunningham, D.J.C. Oxford and Yale physiologists in Colorado in 1911. In *Respiratory control: A modeling perspective*, ed. G. D. Swanson, F. S. Grodins, and R. L. Hughson, 1–9. New York: Plenum, 1989.

Cunningham, D.J.C., and B. B. Lloyd, eds. *The regulation of respiration.* Oxford: Blackwell, 1963.

Dawes, G. S. *Foetal and neonatal physiology,* 53–54. Chicago: Year Book Medical Publishers, 1967.

DeGraff, A. C., Jr., R. F. Grover, R. L. Johnson, J. W. Hammond Jr., and J. M. Miller. Diffusing capacity of the lung in Caucasians native to 3,100 m. *Am. J. Physiol.* 29 (1970): 71–76.

Dill, D. B. A chemical study of certain Pacific Coast fishes. *J. Biol. Chem.* 48 (1921a): 73–82.

———. A chemical study of the California sardine (*Sardinia cærulea*). *J. Biol. Chem.* 48 (1921b): 93–103.

———. *Life, heat, and altitude: Physiological effects of hot climates and high altitudes.* Cambridge, MA: Harvard University Press, 1938.

———. The Harvard Fatigue Laboratory: Its development, contributions, and demise. *Circ. Res.* 20, suppl. 1 (1967): 161–170.

———. Mabel Purefoy FitzGerald: Our second centenarian. *Physiologist* 16 (1973): 247–248.

———. L. J. Henderson, his transition from physical chemist to physiologist, his qualities as a man. *Physiologist* 20 (1977): 1–15.

———. Ten men on a mountain. In *Environmental physiology: Aging, heat, and altitude*, ed. S. M. Horvath and M. K. Yousef, 453–466. New York: Elsiever/North Holland, 1980.

———. Arlie V. Bock, physiologist. *Physiologist* 24 (1981): 11–13.

———. Personal memoirs, unpublished. In possession of David B. Dill Jr.

Dill, D. B., and W. C. Adams. Maximal oxygen uptake at sea level and at 3,090 m altitude in high-school champion runners. *J. Appl. Physiol.* 30 (1971): 854–859.

Dill, D. B., H. T. Edwards, A. Fölling, S. A. Oberg, A. M. Pappenheimer, and J. H. Talbott. Adaptations of the organism to changes in oxygen pressure. *J. Physiol.* 71 (1931): 47–63.

Dill, D. B., W. C. Alexander, L. G. Myhre, J. E. Whinnery, and D. M. Tucker. Aerobic capacity of D. B. Dill. *Fed. Proc.* 44 (1985): 1013.

Donald, K. W. J. S. Haldane's contributions to applied physiology in the armed services, with special reference to diving. In *The regulation of respiration*, ed. D.J.C. Cunningham and B. B. Lloyd, 83–91. Oxford: Blackwell, 1963.

Douglas, C. G. The determination of the total oxygen capacity and blood volume at different altitudes by the carbon monoxide method. *J. Physiol.* 40 (1910): 472–479.

———. *Obituary notices of the Royal Society of London* 2, no. 5 (1936): 115–139. Reprinted in *The regulation of respiration*, ed. D.J.C. Cunningham and B. B. Lloyd, 3–32. Oxford: Blackwell, 1936.

Douglas, C. G., and J. S. Haldane. The causes of absorption of oxygen by the lungs. *J. Physiol.* 44 (1912): 305–354.

Douglas, C. G., J. S. Haldane, and J.B.S. Haldane. The laws of combination of haemoglobin with carbon monoxide and oxygen. *J. Physiol.* 44 (1912): 274–304.

Douglas, C. G., J. S. Haldane, Y. Henderson, and E. C. Schneider. Physiological observations made on Pikes Peak, Colorado, with special reference to adaptation to low barometric pressure. *Phil. Trans. Roy. Soc.* (London) series B 203 (1913): 185–318.

Ellman, R. *Oscar Wilde*. London: Hamish Hamilton, 1987.

FitzGerald, M. P. Three cases of ringworm of the calf transmitted to man. *J. Path. Bacteriol.* (Edinburgh and London) 12 (1908): 232–241.

———. The alveolar carbonic acid pressure in diseases of the blood and in diseases of the respiratory and circulatory systems. *J. Path. Bacteriol.* (Cambridge) 14 (1910a): 328–343.

———. Preliminary note on the origin of the hydrochloric acid in the gastric tubules. *Proc. Roy. Soc.* (London) 82 (1910b): 346–348.

———. The induction of sporulation in the bacilli belonging to 3the *aerogenes capsulatum* group. *J. Path. Bacteriol.* (Cambridge) 15 (1910–1911a): 147–168.

———. The origin of the hydrochloric acid in the gastric tubules. *Proc. Roy. Soc.* (London) 83 (1910–1911b): 56–93.

———. The changes in the breathing and the blood at various high altitudes. *Phil. Trans. Roy. Soc.* (London), series B 203 (1913): 351–371.

———. Further observations on the changes in the breathing and the blood at various high altitudes. *Proc. Roy. Soc.* (London) 88 (1914): 248–258.

FitzGerald, M. P., and J. S. Haldane. The normal alveolar carbonic acid pressure in man. *J. Physiol.* 32 (1905): 486–494.

FitzGerald, M. P., R. I. Whitman, and T.S.P. Strangeways. The value of the opsonic index. *Bull. Com. Study*, spec. dis. (Cambridge, 1907): 115–144.

Fred, H., A. Schmidt, T. Bates, and H. Hecht. Acute pulmonary edema of high altitude: Clinical and physiologic observations. *Circulation* 25 (June 1962): 929–937.

Fulco, C. S., P. B. Rock, and A. Cymerman. Maximal and sub-maximal exercise performance at altitude. *Aviat. Space Environ. Med.* 69 (1998): 793–801.

Glover, G. H., and I. E. Newsom. Brisket disease (dropsy of high altitudes). *Colo. Agr. Exp. Sta. Bul.*, no. 204 (1915): 3–24.

———. Brisket disease (bulletin no. 204, revised) *Colo. Agr. Exp. Sta. Bul.*, no. 229 (1917): 3–8.

———. Further studies on brisket disease. *J. Agricultural Res.* 15 (1918): 409–413.

Gordon, H. H. Community needs and medical school program. (Paper presented at the annual meeting of the alumni of Cornell University Medical College, April 21, 1951.) *Pediatrics* 8 (1951): 841–847.

————. Some methods of improving pediatric care of the newborn. *New York J. Med.* 55 (1955): 2648–2653.

Gordon, H. H., and J. A. Lichty. Colorado premature-infant care program. *Rocky Mtn. Med. J.* 46 (August 1949): 650–652.

Griswold, D. L., and J. H. Griswold. *The history of Leadville and Lake County, Colorado: From mountain solitude to metropolis.* Vol. 6. 1882. Denver: Colorado Historical Society, 1995.

Grollman, A. Letter to Dr. Williams, May 5, and Dr. Williams's reply, May 9. Alan Mason Chesney Medical Archives, Johns Hopkins Medical Institutions, Baltimore, MD, 1923.

————. The combination of phenol red and proteins. *J. Biol. Chem.* 64 (1925): 141–160.

————. The relation of filterable dyes to their excretion and behavior in the animal body. *Am. J. Physiol.* 75 (1926a): 287–293.

————. Ultrafiltration through collodion membranes. *J. Gen. Physiol.* 9 (1926b): 813–826.

————. The effect of variation in posture on the output of the human heart. *Am. J. Physiol.* 86 (1928): 285–301.

————. The urine of the goosefish (*Liphius piscatorius*): Its nitrogenous constituents with special reference to the presence in it of trimethylamine oxide. *J. Biol. Chem.* 81 (1929a): 267–278.

————. The determination of the cardiac output of man by the use of acetylene. *Am. J. Physiol.* 88 (1929b): 432–445.

————. The value of the cardiac output of the normal individual in basal, resting condition. Physiological variations in the cardiac output of man (VI). *Am. J. Physiol.* 90 (1929c): 210–217.

————. Changes in cardiac output, metabolism, blood pressure, and pulse rate of man following the ingestion of fluids. Physiological variations in the cardiac output of man (II). *Am. J. Physiol.* 89 (1929d): 157–162.

————. The effect of high altitude on the cardiac output and its related functions: An account of experiments conducted on the summit of Pikes Peak, Colorado. Physiological variations in the cardiac output of man (VII). *Am. J. Physiol.* 93 (1930a): 19–40.

————. The constancy of the cardiac output from day to day throughout the year. Physiological variations in the cardiac output of man (VIII). *Am. J. Physiol.* 93 (1930b): 536–543.

————. The effect of breathing carbon dioxide and of voluntary forced ventilation on the cardiac output of man. Physiological variations in the cardiac output of man (IX). *Am. J. Physiol.* 94 (1930c): 287–299.

―――. The effect of variations in the environmental temperature on the pulse rate, blood pressure, oxygen consumption, arterio-venous oxygen difference, and cardiac output of normal individuals. Physiological variations in the cardiac output of man (X). *Am. J. Physiol.* 95 (1930d): 263–273.

―――. The pulse rate, blood pressure, oxygen consumption, arterio-venous oxygen difference, and cardiac output of man during normal sleep. Physiological variations in the cardiac output of man (XI). *Am. J. Physiol.* 95 (1930e): 274–284.

―――. The effect of menstrual cycle on the cardiac output, pulse rate, blood pressure, and oxygen consumption of a normal woman. Physiological variations in the cardiac output of man (XII). *Am. J. Physiol.* 96 (1931a): 1–7.

―――. The effect of mild muscular exercise on the cardiac output. Physiological variations in the cardiac output of man (XIII). *Am. J. Physiol.* 96 (1931b): 8–15.

―――. *The cardiac output of man in health and disease.* Baltimore, MD: Charles C. Thomas, 1932.

Grollman, A., and J.C.W. Frazer. The osmotic pressure of aqueous solutions of phenol at 30°. *J. Am. Chem. Soc.* 45 (1923): 1705–1710.

―――. The vapor pressure lowering of aqueous sulfuric acid solutions at 25°. *J. Am. Chem. Soc.* 47 (1925): 712–717.

Grollman, A., and E. K. Marshall Jr. The time necessary for rebreathing in a lung-bag system to attain homogenous mixture. *Am. J. Physiol.* 86 (1928): 110–116.

Grover, R. F. Pulmonary hypertension: The price of high living. In *The pulmonary circulation and gas exchange*, ed. W. W. Wagner and E. K. Weir, 317–341. Armonk, NY: Futura Publishing, 1994.

Gtover, R.F., ed. *Normal and abnormal pulmonary circulation.* Basel, Switzerland: S. Karger, 1963. (Panel discussion on pulmonary edema at high altitude, with C. S. Houston, moderator, and presentations by Hultgren and Visscher, pp. 313–330.)

Grover, R. F., J. T. Reeves, D. H. Will, and S. G. Blount Jr. Pulmonary vasoconstriction in steers at high altitude. *J. Appl. Physiol.* 18 (1963a): 567–574.

Grover, R. F., J.H.K. Vogel, K. H. Averill, and S. G. Blount Jr. Pulmonary hypertension: Individual and species variability relative to vascular reactivity. *Am. Heart J.* 66 (1963b): 1–3.

Grover, R. F., J. T. Reeves, E. B. Grover, and J. E. Leathers. Muscular exercise in young men native to 3,100 m altitude. *J. Appl. Physiol.* 22 (1967): 555–564.

Hackett, P. H., C. E. Creagh, R. F. Grover, B. Honigman, C. S. Houston, J. T. Reeves, A. M. Sophocles, and M. Van Hardenbroek. High-altitude pulmonary edema without the right pulmonary artery. *New Engl. J. Med.* 302, no. 19 (May 8, 1980): 1070–1086.

Haldane, J. S. A letter to Edinburgh professors. London: David Stott, 1890.

———. The action of carbonic acid on man. *J. Physiol.* 18 (1895): 430–462.

———. Investigations on the nature and sources of the suffocative gas met with in wells, together with further observations on the black-damp of coal-mines. *Transactions of the Federal Institution of Mining Engineers* (London) 11 (1896a): 265–273.

———. Report to the secretary of state for the home department on the causes of death in colliery explosions and underground fires, with special reference to the explosions at Tylorstown, Brancepeth, and Micklefield (Cd. 8112). Reports from commissioners, inspectors, and others XVIII (1896b): 611–658.

———. The therapeutic administration of oxygen. *Brit. Med J.* (1917a): 181–183.

———. Organism and environment as illustrated by the physiology of breathing. Silliman Lecture, Yale University Press, 1917b.

Haldane, J. S. Acclimatisation to high altitudes. *Physiol. Rev.* 7 (1927): 363–384.

Haldane, J. S., and R. H. Makgill. The spontaneous combustion of hay. *Fuel in Science and Practice* 2 (1923): 380–387.

Haldane, J. S., and J. L. Smith. The oxygen tension of arterial blood. *J. Physiol.* 20 (1896): 497–517.

Haldane, J. S., and J. G. Priestley. The regulation of the lung ventilation. *J. Physiol.* 32 (1905): 225–266.

———. *Respiration.* 2d ed. New Haven, CT: Yale University Press, 1935.

Haldane, J.B.S. The scientific work of J. S. Haldane (1860–1936). *Nature* 187 (1960): 102–105.

Haldane, L. K. *Friends and kindred.* New York: Faber and Faber, 1961.

Hamilton, W. F. Measurement of cardiac output. In *Circulation*, ed. W. F. Hamilton and P. Dow, vol. 1, sec. 2, 551–584. Washington, DC: American Physiological Society, 1962.

Hansen, J. E., II. *Democracy's college in the Centennial State: A history of Colorado State University.* Salt Lake City, UT: Publisher's Press, 1977.

Hartridge, H., and F.J.W. Roughton. A method of measuring the velocity of very rapid chemical reactions. *Proc Roy Soc.* (London), series A 104 (1923): 376–430.

Havil, W. H., J. A. Lichty Jr., G. B. Taylor, and G. H. Whipple. Renal threshold for hemoglobin in dogs uninfluenced by mercury poisoning (II). *J. Exper. Med.* 55 (1932a): 617–625.

Havil, W. H., J. A. Lichty Jr., and G. H. Whipple. Tolerance for mercury poisoning increased by frequent hemoglobin injections (III). *J. Exper. Med.* 55 (1932b): 627–635.

Hecht, H. H., R. L. Lange, W. H. Carnes, H. Kuida, and J. T. Blake. Brisket disease. *Tr. Assoc. Am. Physicians* 72 (1959): 157.

Henderson, Y. *Adventures in respiration.* Baltimore, MD: Williams and Wilkins, 1938.

Hill, A. V., C.N.H. Long, and H. Lupton. Muscular exercise, lactic acid, and the supply and utilization of oxygen, parts 7–8. *Proc. Roy. Soc.* (London) 97 (1924): 155–167.

Horvath, S. M., and E. C. Horvath. *The Harvard Fatigue Laboratory: Its history and contributions.* Englewood Cliffs, NJ: Prentice Hall, 1973.

———. Twenty-third president: David Bruce Dill (1891–1986). *Physiologist* 30 (1987): 84–85.

Houston, C. S. Pneumonia or heart failure? *Summit* 6 (April 1960a): 2–3.

———. Acute pulmonary edema of high altitude. *New Engl. J. Med.* 263 (10), (Sept. 8, 1960b): 478–480.

———. Letter to Robert F. Grover, March 1999.

Houston, C. S., ed. *High-altitude physiology study.* Collected papers. Published by Arctic Institute of North America; printed by Queen City Printers, Burlington, VT, 1982.

Houston, C. S., and R. H. Bates. *K2: The savage mountain.* London: Collins, 1955.

Houston, C. S., A. Cymerman, and J. R. Sutton. *Operation Everest II.* Natick, MA: U.S. Army Research Institute of Environmental Medicine, 1991.

Howard, R. C., J. A. Lichty, and P. D. Bruns. Measurement of birth weight, body length, and head size. Studies of babies born at high altitude (II). *Am. J. Dis. Child.* 93 (1957a): 670–674.

Howard, R. C., P. D. Bruns, and J. A. Lichty. Arterial oxygen saturation and hematocrit values at birth. Studies of babies born at high altitude (III). *Am. J. Dis. Child.* 93 (1957b): 674–678.

Hsia, C.C.C.W., L. F. Herazo, M. Ramanathan, and R. L. Johnson Jr. Cardiac output during exercise measured by acetylene rebreathing, thermodilution, and Fick techniques. *J. Appl. Physiol.* 78 (1995): 1612–1616.

Hultgren, H. N. *High-altitude medicine.* Stanford, CA: Hultgren Publications, 1997.

Hultgren, H. N., and W. Spickard. Medical experiences in Peru. *Stanford Med. Bull.* 18 (May 1960): 76–95.

Hultgren, H. N., W. B. Spickard, K. Hellriegel, and C. S. Houston. High-altitude pulmonary edema. *Medicine* 40, no. 3 (September 1961): 289–313.

Hultgren, H. N., C. E. Lopez, E. Lundberg, and H. Miller. Physiologic studies of pulmonary edema at high altitude. *Circulation* 24 (March 1964): 393–408.

Hultgren, H. N., R. F. Grover, and L. H. Hartley. Abnormal circulatory responses to high altitude in subjects with a previous history of high-altitude pulmonary edema. *Circulation* 44 (1971): 759–769.

Hultgren, H. N., R. Wilson, and J. C. Kosek. Lung pathology in high-altitude pulmonary edema. *Wilderness Environ. Med.* 8 (1997): 218–220.

Hurtado, A., T. Velásquez, C. Reynafarje, R. Lozano, R. Chávez, H. Aste-Salazar, B. Reynafarje, C. Sánchez, and J. Muñoz. Mechanisms of natural acclimatization: Studies on the native resident of Morococha, Peru, at an altitude of 14,900 feet. Report no. 56-1, 1–62. USAF School of Aviation Medicine, Randolph AFB, TX, 1956.

Jacobs, R., J. S. Robinson, J. A. Owens, J. Falconer, and M.E.D. Webster. The effect of prolonged hypobaric hypoxia on growth of fetal sheep. *J. Dev. Physiol.* 10 (1988): 97–112.

Jensen, G. M., and L. G. Moore. The effect of altitude and other risk factors on birth weight: Independent or interactive effects? *Am. J. Pub. Health* 87 (1997): 1003–1007.

Jensen, R. Right heart failure. *California Veterinarian* 5 (1952): 18–19.

Johnson, R. L., Jr. Letter to Arthur P. Grollman, September 5, 1994.

———. Letter to John T. Reeves, November 3, 1998.

Johnson, R. L., W. S. Spicer, J. M. Bishop, and R. E. Forster. Pulmonary capillary blood volume, flow, and diffusing capacity during exercise. *J. Appl. Physiol.* 15 (1960): 893–902.

Jovanovic, L., A. Kessler, and C. M. Peterson. Human maternal and fetal response to graded exercise. *J. Appl. Physiol.* 58 (1985): 1719–1722.

Kinsman, J. M., J. W. Moore, and W. F. Hamilton. Injection method: Physical and mathematical consideration. Studies on the circulation (I). *Am. J. Physiol.* 89 (1929): 322–330.

Krogh, A., and J. Lindhard. Measurements of blood flow through the lungs of man. *Skand. Arch. Physiologie* 27 (1912): 100–125.

LaBelle, J. C. High-altitude anecdotes. *Canadian Alpine J.* (1972). Reprinted in Houston, C. S., ed., *High Altitude Physiology Study* (1982): 43–48.

Lichty, J. A., Jr. Relation of streptococci antifibrolysin to acute rheumatic fever. *Am. J. Dis. Child.* 62 (1941): 92–100.

————. Well child supervision. *Rocky Mtn. Med. J.* 48 (1951): 344–348.

Lichty, J. A., Jr., and P. D. Bruns. Deaths of unborn infants in Colorado. *Rocky Mtn. Med. J.* 52 (1955): 892–895.

Lichty, J. A., Jr., W. H. Havill, and G. H. Whipple. Renal thresholds for hemoglobin in dogs (I). *J. Exper. Med.* 55 (1932): 603–615.

Lichty, J. A., Jr., R. Y. Ting, P. D. Bruns, and E. Dyar. Incidence of prematurity higher at high altitude. *Public Health Reports* 70 (1955): 230.

————. Relation of altitude to birthweight. Studies of babies born at high altitude (I). *Am. J. Dis. Child.* 93 (1957): 666–669.

Lizzárraga, M. L. Soroche agudo: Edema agudo del pulmon. *Anal. Fac. Med.* (Lima) 38 (1955): 244–274.

Lotgering, F. K., R. D. Gilbert, and L. D. Longo. The interactions of exercise and pregnancy: A review. *Am. J. Obstet. Gynecol.* 149 (1984): 560–568.

Lubchenco, L. O. Personal communication to John T. Reeves, January 8, 1998.

Lubchenco, L. O., C. Hansman, M. Dressler, and E. Boyd. Intrauterine growth as estimated from live-born birth-weight data at twenty-five to forty-two weeks of gestation. *Pediatrics* 32 (1963): 793–800.

Lubchenco, L. O., D. T. Searls, and J. V. Brazie. Neonatal mortality rate: Relationship to birth weight and gestational age. *J. Ped.* 81 (1972): 814–822.

Macht, D. I., A. Grollman, and O. R. Hyndman. Relation between chemical structure of bile acids and their effect on animal and plant tissues. *Am. J. Physiol.* 68 (1924): 141.

Marshall, E. K., Jr. The cardiac output of the normal unanesthetized dog. Studies on the cardiac output of the dog (I). *J. Am. Physiol.* 77 (1926): 459.

————. Cardiac output of man. In *Harvey Lectures*, 57–76, 1929–1930.

————. Autobiographical notes. Alan Mason Chesney Medical Archives, Johns Hopkins Medical Institutions, Baltimore, MD, 1952.

Marshall, E. K., Jr., and A. Grollman. A method for the determination of the circulatory minute volume in man. *Am. J. Physiol.* 86 (1928): 117–137.

Marshall, E. K., Jr., G. A. Harrop, and A. Grollman. The use of nitrogen for determining the circulatory minute volume. *Am. J. Physiol.* 86 (1928): 99–109.

Mayr, E. This is biology. Cambridge, MA: Harvard University Press, 1997.

McGuire, J. D., and J. E. Hansen II. *Chiron's time: A history of the College of Veterinary Medicine and Biomedical Sciences at Colorado State University.* Endowment Fund, Fort Collins, CO, 1983.

Medawer, P. Review of *JBS: The life and works of J.B.S. Haldane*, by Ronald Clark. *New York Review of Books*, October 10, 1968.

Meyer, M. B. Effects of maternal smoking and altitude on birth weight and gestation. In *The epidemiology of prematurity*, 81–104. National Institute of Child Health and Human Development. Baltimore, MD: Urban and Schwarzenberg, 1977.

Miescher-Rusch, F. Bemerkungen zur Lehre von den Atembewegungen. *Arch. Anat. Physiol. Liepzig.* 6 (1885): 355–380.

Monge-M., C. Enfermedad de los Andes: Estudios fisiológicas. *Annal. Fac. Med.* (Lima) 11 (1928): 1–75.

Moore, L. G. Maternal O_2 transport and fetal growth in Colorado, Peru, and Tibet high-altitude residents. *Am. J. Hum. Biol.* 2 (1990): 627–638.

Moore, L. G., D. Jahnigen, S. S. Rounds, J. T. Reeves, and R. F. Grover. Maternal hyperventilation helps preserve arterial oxygenation during high-altitude pregnancy. *J. Appl. Physiol.* 52 (1982a): 690–694.

Moore, L. G., S. S. Rounds, D. Jahnigen, R. F. Grover, and J. T. Reeves. Infant birth weight is related to maternal arterial oxygenation at high altitude. *J. Appl. Physiol.* 52 (1982b): 695–699.

Moore, L. G., D. W. Hershey, D. Jahnigen, and W. Bowes. The incidence of pregnancy-induced hypertension is increased among Colorado residents of high altitude. *Am. J. Ob. Gyn.* 144 (1982c): 423–429.

Moore, L. G., P. Brodeur, O. Chumbe, J. D'Brot, S. Hofmeister, and C. Monge. Maternal hypoxic ventilatory response, ventilation, and infant birth weight at 4300 m. *J. Appl. Physiol.* 60 (1986): 1401–1406.

Motley, H. L., A. Cournand, L. Werko, A. Himmelstein, and D. Dresdale. The influence of short periods of induced acute anoxia upon pulmonary artery pressures in man. *Am. J. Physiol.* 150 (1947): 315–320.

Newsom I. E. Cardiac insufficiency at high altitude. *Am. J. Vet. Med.* 10 (1915): 837–893.

————. Coccidiosis in cattle. *Veterinary Med.* (October 1929): 16–18.

Nicholas, R., P. D. O'Mera, and N. Calonge. Is syncope related to moderate altitude exposure? *J. Am. Med. Assoc.* 268 (1992): 904–906.

Niermeyer, S., E. M. Shaffer, E. Thilo, C. Corbin, and L. G. Moore. Arterial oxygenation and pulmonary arterial pressure in healthy neonates and infants at high altitude. *J. Pediatr.* 123 (1993): 767–772.

Novy, M. J., E. S. Peterson, and J. Metcalfe. Respiratory characteristics of maternal and fetal blood in cyanotic heart disease. *Am. J. Obstet. Gynecol.* 100 (1968): 821–828.

Ounsted, M., V. A. Moar, and A. Scott. Risk factors associated with small-for-date and large-for-date infants. *Br. J. Obstet. Gynaecol.* 92 (1985): 226–232.

Palmer, S. K., S. Zamudio, C. Coffin, S. Parker, E. Stamm, and L. G. Moore. Quantitative estimation of human uterine artery blood flow and pelvic blood flow redistribution in pregnancy. *Obstet. Gynecol.* 80 (1992): 1000–1006.

Passmore, R. J. S. Haldane and industrial medicine. In *The regulation of respiration,* ed. D.J.C. Cunningham and B. B. Lloyd, 93–102. Oxford: Blackwell, 1963.

Peake, O. B. *The Colorado range cattle industry.* Glendale, CA: Arthur Clarke, 1937.

Pembrey, M. S., and R. W. Allen. Observations upon Cheyne Stokes' respiration. *J. Physiol.* 32 (1905): 18P–20P.

Pierson, R. E., and R. Jensen. Brisket disease. In *Diseases of cattle.* Evanston, IL: American Veterinary Publications, 1956.

Pryor, R., W. F. Weaver, and S. G. Blount Jr. Electrocardiographic observation of 493 residents living at high altitude (10,150 feet). *Am. J. Cardiol.* 16 (1965): 494–499.

Pugh, L.G.C.E. Physiological and medical aspects of the Himalayan scientific and mountaineering expedition, 1960–61. *Brit. Med. J.* 2 (1962): 621–627.

Ray G. Daggs Award. *Physiologist* 29 (1986): 55.

Reeves, J. T., R. F. Grover, and J. E. Cohn. Regulation of ventilation during exercise at 10,200 ft in athletes born at low altitude. *J. Appl. Physiol.* 22 (1967): 546–554.

Rennie, D. Herb Hultgren in Peru: What causes high-altitude pulmonary edema? In *Hypoxia into the next millenium,* ed. R. C. Roach, P. D. Wagner, and P. H. Hackett, 1–22. New York: Kluwer Academic/Plenum Publishers, 1999.

Saltin, B., R. F. Grover, C. G. Blomqvist, H. Hartley, and R. L. Johnson. Maximal oxygen uptake and cardiac output after two weeks at 4300 m. *J. Appl. Physiol.* 25 (1968): 400–409.

Schmidt-Nielsen, B. *August and Marie Krogh: Lives in science.* Oxford: Oxford University Press, 1995.

Schoene, R. B., E. R. Swenson, C. J. Pizzo, P. H. Hackett, R. C. Roach, W. J. Mills Jr., W. R. Henderson Jr., and T. R. Martin. The lung at high altitude: Bronchoalveolar lavage in acute mountain sickness and pulmonary edema. *J. Appl. Physiol.* 64 (1988): 2605–2613.

Shime, J., E.J.M. Mocarski, D. Hastings, G. D. Webb, and R. McLaughlin. Congenital heart disease in pregnancy: Short- and long-term implications. *Am. J. Obstet. Gynecol.* 156 (1987): 313–322.

Silverman, W. A. Commentary: Low birth weight. *Pediatrics* 32 (1963): 791–792.

Smith, J. L., and J. S. Haldane. The causes of absorption of oxygen by the lungs. *J. Physiol.* 21 (1897): xvi.

Smith, J. M. Introduction in J.B.S. Haldane's *On being the right size and other essays,* ed. J. M. Smith. Oxford: Oxford University Press, 1985.

Sutton, J. R. Charles Snead Houston. In *Hypoxia, the Adaptations,* ed. J. R. Sutton, G. Coates, and J. E. Remmers, xxv–xxxii. Burlington, ON, Canada: B. C. Dekker, 1990.

Taylor, E. S. Letter to Robert F. Grover, June 21, 1997.

Taylor, E. S., and H. Gordon. The premature-infant program in Colorado. *American Committee on Maternal Welfare Quarterly Bulletin* 10, no. 1 (October 1948): 1–7.

Torrance, R. W. Mabel's normalcy. *J. Medical Biography* 7 (1999): 151–165.

Torre-Bueno, J. R., P. D. Wagner, H. A. Saltzman, G. E. Gale, and R. E. Moon. Diffusion limitation in normal humans during exercise at sea level and simulated altitude. *J. Appl. Physiol.* 58 (1985): 989–995.

Triebwaser, J. H., R. L. Johnson Jr., R. P. Burpo, J. C. Campbell, W. C. Reardon, and C. G. Blomqvist. Noninvasive determination of cardiac output by a modified acetylene rebreathing procedure utilizing mass spectrometer measurements. *Aviat. Space Environ. Med.* 48 (1977): 203–209.

Verbanck, S., H. Larsen, D. Linnarsson, G. K. Prisk, J. B. West, and M. Paiva. Pulmonary tissue volume, cardiac output, and diffusing capacity in sustained microgravity. *J. Appl. Physiol.* 83 (1997): 810–816.

Von Euler, U. S., and G. Liljestrand. Observations on the pulmonary arterial pressure in the cat. *Acta Physiol. Scand.* 12 (1946): 301–320.

Wagner, P. D., G. E. Gale, R. E. Moon, J. R. Torre-Bueno, B. W. Stolp, and H. A. Saltzman. Pulmonary gas exchange in humans exercising at sea level and simulated altitude. *J. Appl. Physiol.* 61 (1986): 260–270.

Wagner, P. D., J. R. Sutton, J. T. Reeves, A. Cymerman, B. M. Groves, and M. K. Malconian. Operation Everest II: Pulmonary gas exchange during a simulated ascent of Mt. Everest. *J. Appl. Physiol.* 63 (1987): 2348–2359.

Warburg, O., and E. Negelein. Über das Absorptionsspektrum des Atmungsferments. *Biochem. Z.* 214 (1929): 64–100.

Watson, J. D. *The double helix.* London: Weidenfeld and Nicolson, 1968.

West, J. B. Diffusing capacity of the lung for carbon monoxide at high altitude. *J. Appl. Physiol.* 17 (1962): 421–426.

———. Strength and failure of pulmonary capillaries. In *The pulmonary circulation and gas exchange,* ed. W. W. Wagner and E. K. Weir, 1–17. Armonk, NY: Futura Publishing, 1994.

Will, D. H., A. F. Alexander, J. T. Reeves, and R. F. Grover. High altitude–induced pulmonary hypertension in normal cattle. *Circulation Res.* 10 (1962): 172–177.

Will, D. H., J. L. Hicks, C. S. Card, and A. F. Alexander. Inherited susceptibility of cattle to high-altitude pulmonary hypertension. *J. Appl. Physiol.* 38 (1975): 491–494.

Williams, L., M. A. Spence, and S. C. Tiedeman. Implications of the observed effect of air pollution on birth weight. *Social Biology* 24, no. 1 (1977): 1–10.

World Health Organization. Manual of international statistical classification of diseases, injuries, and causes of death. Adopted 1948. Geneva: WHO, 1949.

———. Recommendations regarding statistics of perinatal and maternal deaths. ICD9 Rev. Conf. 75.24, Rev. 1, Annex II. Geneva: WHO, 1975.

Zamudio, S., S. K. Palmer, T. Droma, E. Stamm, C. Coffin, and L. G. Moore. Effect of altitude on uterine artery blood flow during normal pregnancy. *J. Appl. Physiol.* 79 (1995a): 7–14.

Zamudio, S., S. K. Palmer, T. E. Dahms, J. Berman, T. Droma, R. G. McCullough, R. E. McCullough, and L. G. Moore. Alterations in uteroplacental blood flow precede hypertension in preeclampsia at high altitude. *J. Appl. Physiol.* 79 (1995b): 15–22.

Zuntz, N., A. Loewy, A. F. Mueller, and W. Caspari. *Höhenklima und Bergwanderungen in ihrer Wirkung auf den Menschen.* Berlin: Bong, 1860.

INDEX

Page numbers in italics indicate illustrations.